Linguistic Theory for Aphasia

Maria Garraffa • Giuditta Smith

Linguistic Theory for Aphasia

palgrave
macmillan

Maria Garraffa
Faculty of Medicine and Health sciences
University of East Anglia
Norwich, UK

Giuditta Smith
Faculty of Medicine and Health sciences
University of East Anglia
Norwich, UK

ISBN 978-3-031-77133-0   ISBN 978-3-031-77134-7   (eBook)
https://doi.org/10.1007/978-3-031-77134-7

This Palgrave Macmillan imprint is published by the registered company Springer Nature Switzerland AG.
The registered company address is: Gewerbestrasse 11, 6330 Cham, Switzerland

If disposing of this product, please recycle the paper.

PREFACE

Establishing a direct link between linguistics and aphasia is a complex endeavor due to the heterogeneous nature of the language disorder in individuals with aphasia, and the descriptive nature of linguistic theory often idealizing language competence. Furthermore, the manifestation of a language disorder in people with aphasia quite often stems from strategic linguistic behaviors developed by the speaker to respond to a challenging communicative task, rather than a true reflection of the language ability. From a linguistic standpoint, aphasia presents a multifaceted phenomenon where all levels of linguistic analysis are pertinent to its investigation. The severity of aphasia ranges from a complete lack of language capacities to milder impairments that offer insights into the linguistic operations required, for instance, to produce complex sentences.

Complicating matters further, language is intricately intertwined with ancillary cognitive functions such as memory, attention, emotions, and sensory processing. This interconnectedness underscores the inadequacy of linguistic analysis in isolation to fully describe the language impairment in aphasia, hindering both accurate diagnosis and effective treatment.

Ruth Lesser's seminal work in 1978 marked the first systematic discussion of the contributions of linguistics to the study of aphasia. Lesser emphasized the pivotal role of linguistic descriptions of language disorders in contrast to a purely medical approach focused on physical improvement, diagnostic labeling, and formulaic language usage for functional communication. Lesser's book presents a rich set of linguistics terminology and a framework covering each linguistics aspect (semantics, syntax, and phonology).

Despite advancements in both linguistics and aphasiology, efforts to foster dialogue between the disciplines have been insufficient, leading to missed opportunities for enhancing our understanding of language disorders in aphasia. However, linguistics-based tools are indispensable for evaluating the language of individuals with aphasia and delving into the underlying reasons for language impairments.

This book aims to offer a short overview of some linguistic concepts applied to the study of aphasic language disorders and their contributions to detailed language investigation and intervention planning. While not exhaustive, it serves as a catalyst for collaboration between clinical and linguistic programs, encouraging the development of a shared framework to address the complexities posed by individuals with aphasia. Through interdisciplinary cooperation, we can better navigate the dilemmas and challenges inherent in understanding and treating aphasic language disorders, but this requires sharing some of the specific terminology across fields educating future practitioners to formulate targets informed by linguistic theories. This is our aim; this is our hope.

The authors.

Norwich, UK   Maria Garraffa
                                                                           Giuditta Smith

CONTENTS

LIST OF FIGURES

LIST OF TABLES

CHAPTER 1

Introduction

Abstract Which are the common principles in aphasiology that can facilitate the integration of linguistics in the assessment and treatment of people with aphasia? How can linguistics support a better investigation of the language in people with aphasia? Is linguistics necessary for language assessment and therapy in people with aphasia or can diagnosis and therapeutical targets be set without referring to linguistics components and within non-linguistics models? This chapter is a brief overview on the influence of linguistic theory for aphasiology, covering foundation concepts of the field of aphasiology from an historical point of view. It will briefly summarize the main topics of the book and propose points for discussion on the general link between linguistics and aphasia, discussing the implications of generating predictions based on the theory of language to better understand the language profile and the needs of people with aphasia.

Keywords Fractionation assumption • Associations • Dissociations • Transparency/subtractivity assumption

1.1   Linguistics and Aphasia: Some Assumptions

Aphasia does not manifest as a single disorder, and it can be approached as a complex cluster of language-based conditions with effects on the language faculty and visible in its modalities, for example production and comprehension. There is much variation in how it manifests itself, in both its severity and its recovery. The variation of the language impairment in people with aphasia makes the contribution from linguistics crucial to navigate the heterogeneity of the language disorders as it provides a theoretic tool to systematize the language disorder, and to create predictions for treatments and recovery in general. Traditional neurological classifications and psycholinguistics models have not often been able to explain aphasic syndromes and a collection of a detailed language profile represents the core part of the work for both researchers and therapists working with people with aphasia. The challenges for aphasiology are thus about the integration of information coming from different disciplines with a methodological approach that is divisive with language profile and neurological diagnoses not "talking the same language."

One of the most fundamental assumptions that has driven the development of neuropsychology of language has been the so-called *fractionation assumption* (Caramazza, 1984; see Coltheart, 2017 for a more recent overview). This approach was developed in neuropsychology to isolate the language components (lexicon, phonology, semantics, syntax) in the brain and make use of these isolated modules as generators of research questions for the investigation of aphasia language disorders. Research supportive of the fractionation assumption investigates a specific language component, for example verbs in a naming task, or verbs in a comprehension task, to establish if an impairment on verbs is selective for production and does not occur in comprehension, or if word retrieval in a person with aphasia is disturbed due to a semantic impairment or to a phonological impairment. This methodological assumption requires that a language-based cognitive function, for example verb naming or semantic vs. phonological word retrieval, can be described in a model and represented in the brain in isolation and, more importantly, with some sort of biological evidence in support of the "location" dedicated to the individual components proposed in the model. According to the fractionation assumption, different language functions in the brain represent the optimal testing ground for the investigation of a cognitive model of language, and people with brain lesions provide evidence for discerning which component or module of the system is disrupted in people aphasia. This has been discussed in classic literature also as related to the *transparency condition* (Caramazza, 1984) or to the *subtractivity assumption* (Saffran, 1982): in a patient with brain damage, a module can be subtracted from the general modular system, and the reduced system can be investigated as the result of this subtraction. One of the main assumptions of the transparency condition model is that the cognitive system of a person with aphasia does not undergo a reorganization of the unimpaired components or the creation of new modules to cope with the neurological disruption. The implication of the transparency/subtractivity assumption is that the process involved in the language function preonset is not affected by the language disruption and it does not work differently. Otherwise, the language recorded by the speech and language therapists would be a strategic adaptation to a new system, instead of a genuine profile of the language system itself, and the pathological performance would not have a transparent relation to the processing of a typical language system, making the analysis of pathological cases irrelevant for the understanding of normal cognition. The main empirical methodology often adopted in neuropsychology for justifying the fractionation assumption is the established view that language functions are dissociable in aphasia and, more importantly, that dissociations can be discovered in relation to other functions, double dissociations. Over a century of research in aphasia has documented, if nothing else, that brain damage can result in differentiated patterns of language impairments: some patients present with marked difficulties in one area, for example in naming verbs, in the context of otherwise spared language functions; other patients present a different constellation of spared and impaired language functions, for example an impairment in naming across both grammatical categories but not for concrete nouns. While an interesting and elegant observation, it does not tell much about the reason for these distinctions and the possible mechanisms that can justify these distinctions, first in the language system and then in the brain. A necessary part of the theoretical and empirical development of cognitive neuropsychology is the formulation of coherent categories of aphasia that are defined in a framework of natural language function, which is not possible to formulate without a linguistics analysis. This implies that aphasic symptoms should be defined not in terms of the "pre-theoretical" symptoms such as comprehension and repetition disorder, or with a mixed vocabulary such as "posterior aphasia with spared comprehension," but in terms of categories that are derived from a theoretically defensible model of language.

In this book, we propose an approach that defines aphasia as a language disorder resulting from a neurological event. A simple term, such as aphasia, provides an open framework that can then be specified by a set of inferences based on linguistic distinctions attested in natural languages and to integrate the context of use of a language and its sociolinguistics consequences, often neglected in the study of language in people with aphasia. The focus will then be on the application of linguistics to language disorders in aphasia and less on the neurological consequences of a brain damage, although some aspect of the brain activity, such as the response to brain stimulation, will be relevant and discussed in the final chapter.

1.2   Is Linguistics Necessary for the Investigation of Language in Aphasia?

In the last century, starting from Jakobson's (1956) investigation of aphasia, many linguistically informed approaches to aphasia have emerged, which are aimed at describing and characterizing language impairment. Jakobson proposed that two fundamental operations could be affected in aphasia: the *selection* of lexical items; and the *combination* of these items in linguistically meaningful units. For example, the meaning of a sentence such as "They are sleeping" is computed based on the lexical items selected during a first operation (They, not just one; sleeping, not resting; are, not is) and, subsequently, based on the relative ordering of these lexical items (*They are sleeping*; not *Sleeping are they*), which is the second fundamental operation. According to Jakobson's model, selective disorders of these two operations lead to two distinct types of aphasia: selection aphasia (for example, as a word-finding problem) and combination aphasia (as in agrammatism). Jakobson's intuition that aphasia can be studied and characterized by making use of insights and concepts/notions from linguistics paved the way for many linguistically informed studies on aphasia and the two proposed operations, selection and combination, can be easily recognized in both theoretical models and clinical intervention.

Jakobson's approach is based on the idea that aphasia is a medical term and "it is linguists who have to tell us what the exact nature is of this diverse disintegration." At that time, however, it was difficult to convince linguists to look at the language of people with aphasia, as this is often very fragmented and not as rich as typical language. The consequence was that the first case studies investigated by linguists were not representative of the clinical population, recording and analyzing many fluent speakers and highly educated people with fluent aphasia. A step ahead for the integration of linguistics in the study of the aphasic language was the formulation of linguistics as an approach to investigate language as a mental process. This occurred with the development of transformational grammar by Chomsky (Chomsky, 1957, 1965) and the start of a new discipline: psycholinguistics. One problem that emerged soon after was the need for a systematic mapping of lesions in aphasia and language functions, shifting the interest from linguistics analyses to neurolinguistics mapping, i.e., the anatomical correlates of language and their precise localization in the brain. The increasing interest in mapping specific grammatical operations in brain territories have created some remarkably interesting proposals and very detailed research programs, as was detailed, for example, in the *Syntacto-Topic Conjecture* (Grodzinsky & Friederici, 2006; Grodzinsky, 2006), which stated that:

(a) Major syntactic operations are neurologically individuated.
(b) The organization of these operations in brain space is linguistically significant.

This model made the strong assumption that what we see in language is mapped in the brain, with a clear call for a full integration of linguistics in aphasiology.

The blending of linguistics theories with neurological data and psychological techniques is not a trivial matter. In Britain, the importance of linguistics for studying language disorders has been acknowledged and included in training speech and language therapists; but this is not always the case in other countries. Detailed linguistics investigations of the language of people with aphasia are often either not covered in linguistics programs, or they are just mentioned as an argument for the modularity of specific language components in the brain. Medicine programs do not offer elements of clinical linguistics in their programs, with the exception of the Speech and Language Therapy (SLT) curricula that is taught uniquely to SLTs (Speech and Language Therapists). Linguistics has not yet engaged in a full dialogue with medicine, despite the fact that, in the assessment of several cognitive disorders, language behavior is at the center of many core symptoms (see, for example, the case of pragmatics for ASD [Autistic Spectrum Disorder] or ADHD [Attention Deficit Hyperactivity Disorder]).

Considering this conversation between linguistics and medicine as a tension between a neurological description of aphasia and/or a linguistic profile of it, there are a few important milestones that cannot be ignored.

First, language cannot be quantified just in terms of a single empirical dimension (for example, a temporal dimension or a spatial dimension). Language is not a uniform set of data, and it is not always the case that collecting a two-minute speech sample is more efficient than collecting a shorter sample, or that collecting 40 words is less effective for profiling language than collecting 100 words. Even the mean length utterance (MLU), a frequently used measure of expressive language ability, is often not very revealing if applied to the clinical setting or compared to other linguistics-informed measures, such as number of different words or tense accuracy (Dethorne et al., 2005). MLU has been reported as being impacted by non-linguistic factors, as well as not mirroring any theory of language acquisition where links between, for example, semantic and morphosyntactic development emerge not from a unitary cognitive mechanism but from the interlinked relation of one language domain to another. As an example, Language acquisition data have reported that knowledge of one language domain such as syntax can be "bootstrapped" from another domain, such as phonology. Knowing the meaning of a word can imply that the speaker knows about its syntactic properties, and knowledge about syntax can facilitate acquisition of word meaning (Gleitman & Gleitman, 1992). We will look at this point in detail in the chapter about syntactic impairment in aphasia and its intricate relation with semantics.

Another remarkable contribution of linguistics in the investigation of language in aphasia is the establishment of distinct levels of analyses that cannot be defined simplistically in terms of modalities (production vs. comprehension), but are theoretically-informed and can propose a different point of view in the investigation of the aphasic language. The conventional approach is to consider at least four levels: the sound system (phonology); the system of meanings (semantics); the combinatorial structural organization (syntax); and the coherent use of narratives (pragmatics). In this book we will also include a more detailed level for words (morphology) as the internal structure of the word has been the subject of several investigations into aphasia. Table 1.1 provides the linguistics-based

Table 1.1 Linguistic components, topics and associated terminology covered in the book

Linguistic components	Selected topics	Essential terminology
Phonology	Complexity in phonological errors	Sonority principle
	Effective phonological based therapy	Syllabic clusters
		Phonological markedness
Morphology	Word composition	Derivation
	Morphological derivation	Inflection
	Word classes	Affix
	Training in lexical retrieval	Grammatical class
Semantics	Semantic knowledge in lexical retrieval	Semantic features
	Use of pronouns	Reference
	Predicates	Pronoun resolution
Syntax	Reversible passive	Agreement
	Subject–verb agreement	Intervention
	Relative clauses	Feature
Pragmatics	Abilities in conversations	Implicatures
	Level of text comprehension	Speech acts
	Discourse coherence	Macrostructures
		Microstructures

phenomena selected for each component that we will cover in the current book.

The topics selected in this book do not cover the entire research on clinical linguistics in people with aphasia. They should be considered as evidence on how productive the dialogue between linguistics and aphasia is and as a first step to investigating language within linguistics models and concepts.

It also important to mention that there are several methods for linguistic analysis of spontaneous language, including the Northwestern Narrative Language Analysis system (NNLA, Thompson et al., 1995) and its automation in the CLAN software within the Aphasia Bank (see Fromm et al., 2020). The NNLA is a particular effective tool as it codes grammatical measures (i.e., sentence and verb argument structure) and it is linguistically informed. This area will see more development in the future due to the presence of AI and its application across languages and aphasias (see, for example, a review from Privitera et al., 2024).

1.3   A Note on Rehabilitation of Language in Aphasia

In contemporary aphasia therapy, two primary methodologies prevail: the impairment-based and consequences-based approaches, each with distinct theoretical underpinnings and therapeutic goals.

The impairment-based approach, rooted in cognitive neuropsychology, dissects language into interrelated yet functionally independent modules. By pinpointing the precise locus of functional damage within these modules, therapists can tailor interventions directly to address the specific impairment. This approach, akin to the neurolinguistic perspective, targets the improvement of linguistic deficits resulting from damage to components of the cognitive system.

Conversely, the consequences-based approach, also known as the functional or psychosocial approach, traces its origins to the pragmatic viewpoint, which prioritizes enhancing language use in real-life communication settings. Acknowledging that aphasia not only disrupts language but also profoundly affects individuals' daily lives, this approach emphasizes mitigating the broader consequences of aphasia on social interactions, familial relationships, occupational roles, and societal integration. It aligns closely with the disability model outlined in the World Health Organization's International Classification of Functioning, Disability, and Health (ICF). Over the past several years, these two approaches have frequently been in opposition (see Hillis et al., 2007).

Despite historical tensions between these approaches, efforts to reconcile their differences have emerged. One notable initiative is the book *Aphasia Rehabilitation: The Impairment and Its Consequences* (Martin et al., 2008), where case studies featuring individuals with aphasia are analyzed from both impairment-based and consequences-based perspectives. Through collaborative discourse, the book aims to elucidate the similarities and disparities between these two therapeutic paradigms, fostering a more integrated approach to aphasia intervention. The two approaches are not mutually exclusive, and both require a linguistic-based analysis of the language in people with aphasia, as they both want to reorganize the system of natural language and not support a strategic adaptation to it. This second option will clash very soon with a nonfunctional speaker able to respond to preordered instructions, like an artificial intelligence system working on pre-organized data, but not mastering fully the creative essential component of the natural language.

1.4 Summary

Aphasia is defined as a primary language disorder that manifests itself both neurologically and linguistically as a set of diverse associations and dissociations of language-based symptoms. A language-based description of symptoms is necessary to classify the aphasic disorder, and it must be reported by the person with aphasia as something out of the ordinary on their language abilities that is experienced often with a link to a neurological event. Some of the symptoms can be difficult to assess without linguistics-based assessments, with the risk that the language reported in the spontaneous speech of a person with aphasia will mirror a strategic adaptation for functional communication targets and not the biological manifestation of the impaired function. To avoid misdiagnosis or the neglect of a language disorder in people with aphasia, it is necessary to frame the language-based symptoms manifested in aphasia within natural language models and classify aphasia within linguistic models to formulate informed predictions and therapeutic plans based on the actual function and not based on heuristics externals to the language function.

1.5 Discussion Topics

1. Language in people with aphasia has been investigated within a modular approach based on the impairment of selective functions. Discuss the importance of the fractionation assumption for the development of cognitive models of language and its limitations.
2. The transparency condition has been proposed to integrate linguistic operations within cognitive models. Describe some studies that have used this approach, mentioning the role of dissociations.
3. Associations of language-based symptoms in people with aphasia, for example a deficit in sentence comprehension often associated with a disturbance in thematic mapping, can open a rich ground for therapy. Select one association of language-based symptoms and discuss it in the light of a rehabilitation plan.
4. Two approaches have been proposed in aphasia rehabilitation. Discuss some positives and negatives for both in the light of developing a therapeutical plan to support the natural language system.
5. Discuss the implications of training in linguistics in a medical degree, bringing examples from specialized courses (such as Speech and

Language) but also other programs, for example on language development, ageing or neurodegenerative disorders.
6. The current society is facing a revolution in how we communicate. Discuss aspects of communication relevant for digital health with a particular focus on new opportunities to measure language abilities in speakers with aphasia.

REFERENCES

Caramazza, A. (1984). The logic of neuropsychological research and the problem of patient classification in aphasia. *Brain and Language, 21*(1), 9–20.

Chomsky, N. (1957). Logical structure in language. *Journal of the American Society for Information Science, 8*(4), 284.

Chomsky, N. (1965). Persistent topics in linguistic theory. *Diogenes, 13*(51), 13–20.

Coltheart, M. (2017). The assumptions of cognitive neuropsychology: Reflections on Caramazza (1984, 1986). *Cognitive Neuropsychology, 34*(7–8), 397–402.

Dethorne, Johnson, B. W., & Loeb, J. W. (2005). A closer look at MLU: What does it really measure? *Clinical Linguistics & Phonetics, 19*(8), 635–648.

Fromm, D., MacWhinney, B., & Thompson, C. K. (2020). Automation of the northwestern narrative language analysis system. *Journal of Speech Language and Hearing Research, 63*(6), 1835–1844. https://doi.org/10.1044/2020_JSLHR-19-00267

Gleitman, L. R., & Gleitman, H. (1992). A picture is worth a thousand words, but that's the problem: The role of syntax in vocabulary acquisition. *Current Directions in Psychological Science, 1*, 31–35.

Grodzinsky, Y. (2006). A blueprint for a brain map of syntax. *Broca's region*, 83–107.

Grodzinsky, Y., & Friederici, A. (2006). Neuroimaging of syntax and syntactic processing. *Current Opinion in Neurobiology, 16*(2), 240–246.

Hillis, A., Worrall, L., & Thompson, C. (2007). *The state of impairment-and consequences-based approaches to treatment for aphasia.* In N. Martin, C. Thompson, & L. Worrall (Eds.), *Aphasia rehabilitation: The impairment and its consequences* (pp. 261–271). Plural Publishing.

Jakobson, R. (1956). Two aspects of language and two types of aphasic disturbances. In R. Jakobson & M. Halle (Eds.), *Fundamentals of language* (pp. 115–133). Mouton.

Martin, N., Thompson, C. K., & Worrall, L. (2008). *Aphasia rehabilitation: The impairment and its consequences.* Plural Publishing.

Privitera, A. J., Ng, S. H. S., Kong, A. P. H., & Weekes, B. S. (2024). AI and Aphasia in the Digital Age: A Critical Review. *Brain Sciences, 14*(4), 383.

Saffran, E. M. (1982). Neuropsychological approaches to the study of language. *British Journal of Psychology, 73*(3), 317–337.

Thompson, C. K., Shapiro, L. P., Tait, M. E., Jacobs, B. J., Schneider, S. L., & Ballard, K. J. (1995). A system for the linguistic analysis of agrammatic language production. *Brain and Language, 51*, 124–129.

CHAPTER 2

Disorders of Phonology in Aphasia

Abstract In this chapter, we will explore various aspects of phonological disorders in aphasia. We will examine the concept of phonological complexity and its implications for defining phonological intervention based on data from aphasia research. Our discussion will draw from interdisciplinary studies in aphasia, specifically in relation to generative phonology and the notion of phonological markedness. Additionally, we will showcase a treatment study that focuses on letter–sound correspondence training within a phonological complexity framework based on sonority principle and the format of syllabic clusters. Furthermore, we will touch upon bilingual aphasia and examine the phenomenon of phonological transfer between languages as a relevant factor in understanding phonological disorders.

Keywords Syllabic complexity • Apraxia of speech • Sonority • Pseudowords • Markedness effect

2.1 Introducing Phonology in Aphasia

The frequency of phonetic errors in aphasia serves as a pivotal indicator for clinically classifying patients as either fluent or dysfluent/nonfluent. Dysfluent individuals typically exhibit a significant number of speech errors, while fluent patients tend to demonstrate markedly lower error

M. Garraffa, G. Smith, *Linguistic Theory for Aphasia*,
https://doi.org/10.1007/978-3-031-77134-7_2

13

rates. Given the prominent role of speech problems in defining the language impairment associated with aphasia and devising appropriate intervention strategies, it is crucial to delve deeper into the linguistic underpinnings of these errors.

While various non-language-related factors can influence speech fluency in aphasic patients, our focus here is on elucidating key language-based phonetic errors frequently observed in this population. By leveraging concepts derived from linguistics, we aim to refine the description and understanding of these errors.

Among the notable language-based phonetic errors encountered in aphasia are phonemic paraphasia, where incorrect phonemes are substituted for the intended ones, and perseverations, involving the repetition of previously uttered sounds or syllables. Additionally, phonetic distortions, characterized by alterations in the production of speech sounds, and apraxic errors, stemming from impaired motor planning and execution of speech movements, are common manifestations of aphasic speech disorders.

To enhance our comprehension of these errors, drawing from linguistic frameworks such as phonology and articulatory phonetics can provide valuable insights. Phonological analyses can elucidate the underlying patterns and rules governing the occurrence of specific phonetic errors, while articulatory phonetics offers a detailed examination of the articulatory gestures and mechanisms involved in speech production.

By employing linguistic concepts to refine the description and analysis of phonetic errors in aphasia, we can better tailor intervention strategies to address the unique linguistic challenges faced by individuals with aphasic speech disorders. This interdisciplinary approach fosters a deeper understanding of aphasia and enhances the efficacy of therapeutic interventions aimed at improving speech fluency and communication abilities in affected individuals.

In individuals with aphasia, slow speech arises from both intersyllabic pauses and elongations of consonants and vowels. While aphasic patients tend to make errors in the production of isolated words, such as word repetition, word reading, and picture naming, errors in these tasks are not typically observed in neurotypical speakers. However, when engaged in connected spontaneous speech or experimental settings designed to elicit errors, both aphasic and typical speakers may exhibit errors, albeit in different contexts.

In such conditions, contextual errors predominate, often manifesting as anticipations or perseverations of segments within the utterance, particularly between closely associated content words. These errors reflect a complexity-driven phenomenon, where the linguistic context influences error patterns. Conversely, noncontextually errors tend to stem from simplifications, reflecting a different underlying cognitive process.

Stemberger's research highlights the distinction between contextual and non-contextual errors, emphasizing the tendency for contextual errors to complicate linguistic structures, such as creating complex forms from simple onsets (see Stemberger, 1990, 1991). Understanding these patterns of error production is essential in clinical practice, as they can aid in diagnosing patients' impairments and in monitoring spontaneous recovery and therapeutic progress. By utilizing carefully constructed testing materials that account for linguistic complexity, clinicians can more accurately assess patients' language abilities and tailor interventions accordingly.

Interestingly, influential models of word production, such as those proposed by G. S. Dell and colleagues (e.g., Dell, 1986, 1988), have largely overlooked the effects of linguistic complexity. By integrating insights from research on contextual and noncontextually errors, future models of word production could achieve a more comprehensive understanding of the mechanisms underlying aphasic speech disorders, leading to more effective therapeutic strategies and improved patient outcomes.

Contemporary psycholinguistic models of speech production propose a distinct organization of phonological and phonetic encoding processes. According to these models, an abstract phonological form is initially planned, followed by the encoding of a more detailed phonetic-based motor plan (Levelt, 1989; Levelt et al., 1999). While the specific representations and cognitive processes associated with these encoding stages may vary among models, most accounts agree that phonological encoding involves accessing suprasegmental and segmental representations of a word, including its syllabification.

One key piece of evidence supporting the presence of an abstract phonological representation comes from the observation of phoneme exchange and substitution errors in spontaneous speech errors made by typical speakers (commonly known as slips of the tongue; Fromkin, 1973). For instance, instances where phonemes shift out of their original word positions (such as the /Z/-/n/ exchange in "Noyeux Joël" instead of "Joyeux Noël" for "Happy Christmas") indicate that words are not encoded solely as whole units but that abstract segmental representations

are accessed during speech planning before a specific phonetic plan is for-
mulated. Also, both phonological and phonetic processes are believed to
be influenced by specific linguistic properties, a topic explored further in
the following paragraphs.

Another phenomenon that is pervasive in the research on phonological
errors in people with aphasia is the investigation of reading-aloud patterns
of errors, as in the case of phonological dyslexia. Phonological dyslexia
manifests mainly as impaired reading of pseudowords with the absence of
semantic reading errors; there are usually no errors in reading of real words.

The next section will cover an outline of linguistics principles applied to
the study of phonological errors in people with aphasia.

2.2   Principle of Markedness

Originally intended to categorize specific sound relationships, the concept
of markedness has evolved to encompass various phonological considerations, including characteristics such as commonness, rarity, simplicity,
complexity, early acquisition, and late acquisition. This expansion has
allowed markedness to be applied to a wide range of phonological relationships, aiding in the differentiation of varying degrees of phonological
well-formedness within a language (Goldrick & Daland, 2009;
Hume, 2003).

Within linguistic theory, structures prevalent within individual languages and across different languages are often designated as less marked.
While markedness statements offer valuable insights, they do not fully
address why certain structures deemed "better" (less marked/less complex) exhibit a broader distribution. To truly comprehend the hierarchies
of markedness, one must delve into the underlying factors that contribute
to the widespread distribution of these structures, rather than solely attrib-
uting it to frequency of occurrence. Simply put, understanding what drives
a structure to have a wide distribution is essential for markedness hierarchies to hold significance beyond surface-level affirmations.

It is widely recognized that certain syllable structures, such as the basic
CV pattern, are prevalent across languages and are frequently utilized
within them. Conversely, other types of syllables are comparatively rare
across different languages. Additionally, it is crucial to acknowledge the
principle that if a language encompasses syllables of a certain complexity
level, it will inherently incorporate all simpler types as well (as posited by
Greenberg in Greenberg, 1978). Linguists, leveraging distributional

evidence, have developed hierarchies of syllabic complexity, organizing syllables based on the arrangement of consonants and vowels, known as consonant–vowel templates. Every language contains syllables with a solitary consonant followed by a vowel (CV syllables), with more intricate configurations becoming progressively less common. By considering each variation of the consonant–vowel template as an added layer of complexity, one can construct a hierarchy as follows (based on Clements & Keyser, 1983 and Kaye & Lowenstamm, 1981):

1. Simplest syllabic clusters: CV
2. Intermediate complexity level: CCV, V, CVC
3. More complex clusters: CCCV, CCVC, VC
   – And so forth.

2.3   Syllabic Complexity: The Sonority Principle

In addition, the frequency of syllable types varies within the same consonant–vowel template, depending on which segments make up the syllable. For example, syllables of the format CCV (intermediate level) like /sto/ are more common than syllables like /tle/, although they share the same basic format.

One way to explain this variation of complexity in syllables of the same format is by introducing the distinctions between complex syllables in terms of a principle of **sonority**. In the context of perception, sonority corresponds to the relative loudness of a segment. On the other hand, in the context of production, sonority is defined as the openness of the vocal tract.

Sonority in linguistics is described as the relative measure of intensity or the acoustic energy related to the openness of the vocal tract during speech production (Clements, 1990). Despite the difficulty of defining sonority in more formal terms, there is good agreement in phonology on the relative sonority of different speech sounds. Sonority hierarchies vary somewhat according to which sounds are grouped together. The one presented in Table 2.1 is typical sonority scale.

According to Clement's **Sonority Dispersion Principle** (Clements, 1990), the simplest (more commonly attested in natural languages) syllables are those where there is a maximal, sharp rise in sonority from the edge of the syllable to the peak (the vowel) and little or no decrement

Table 2.1   Sonority scale for the English language, from highest sounds to lowest sounds

Most sonorous to less sonorous	Samples from English language
Low vowels (open vowels)	/a ə/
Mid vowels	/e o/
High vowels (closed vowels)/ glides	/i u /j w/
Flaps	[ɾ]
laterals	/l/
nasals	/m n ŋ/
voiced fricatives	/v ð z/
voiceless fricatives	/f θ s/
voiced plosives	/b d g/
voiceless plosives	/p t k/

afterwards (one example is the syllable /ka/). These syllables produce a cycle with sharp periodic alternations in sonority. On the opposite range, syllables with a flatter profile and no peaks are less preferred as they are prone to sonority dispersion (e.g., /frya/).

Syllable clusters can be ranked according to how well they can be mapped to the optimal sonority profile and this ranking accounts well for differences in frequency of occurrence of syllables in natural languages, even within the same syllable template. For example, within the syllable cluster CV in onset, /da/ is preferred to /la/. Alternatively, in the coda position, /al/ is better than /ad/.

There is evidence this syllabic simplification occurs in natural language, as can be seen through the observation of young children's speech. Many studies have reported a tendency to reduce consonant clusters to a singleton, thus reducing a CCV template to a simpler CV template (Stemberger & Bernhardt, 1997; Ingram, 1974; Smith, 1973; Spencer, 1988). In addition, an elegant study by Ohala (1999) has shown that the simplifications reported in children's speech do follow the rules of the sonority dispersion principle. Of the two consonants, the child will produce the best sonority profile for that syllable. Thus, our young speaker will prefer producing the least sonorous consonant in onset and the most sonorous consonant in coda. These observations are relevant to support the hypothesis that syllabic clusters are based on sonority principles, making a plausible definition of syllabic complexity based on a universal requirement of preserving sonority in sounds' definition.

Complexity plays a significant role in the speech errors of aphasic patients, echoing patterns observed in children's speech development. Multiple studies indicate that aphasic individuals tend to delete consonants more frequently in complex onset environments compared to simple ones. Moreover, aphasic patients exhibit systematic elimination of complex vowel sequences, such as hiatuses, either through consonant epenthesis or vowel deletion, reflecting the notion that sonority serves as a proxy for sound complexity in natural languages.

Taking cues from universal linguistic principles, Romani and Calabrese (1998) conducted an in-depth analysis of errors made by a patient with Broca's aphasia, DB. The authors found a consistent tendency towards sound simplification across the patient's speech, with deletion frequency increasing according to syllable format and the sonority dispersion principle. Deletions primarily affected the most sonorous consonants in complex onsets, aligning with the optimization of syllable sonority profiles predicted by the Sonority Dispersion Principle. Additionally, the use of consonant epenthesis to eliminate hiatuses showcased a strategic approach to managing production complexity.

In a subsequent study by Romani et al. (2002), data from a fluent aphasic patient revealed a lack of simplification tendency, despite similarities with the patient with Broca's aphasia. This discrepancy suggests a potential relationship between articulatory deficits (fluent/nonfluent) and syllabic structure complexity, with nonfluent aphasic speakers showing less susceptibility to complexity effects.

The concept of syllabic complexity driving simplification in aphasia extends to patients with Primary Progressive Aphasia (PPA) aphasia, where phonemic paraphasia often involves transferring marked syllables to more prototypical CV formats (Paradis & Beland, 2002). This universal process is evident not only in aphasic patients but also in second language learners attempting to produce French words, where syllabic errors tend to converge towards simplified formats.

2.4   ASSESSMENT OF PHONOLOGY IN APHASIA

Therapies targeting phonological sequence knowledge have been developed to improve language skills, with some focusing on the phonological properties of words. One such approach, the Phonomotor Therapy (PMT; Kendall & Nadeau, 2016), emphasizes training individual phonemes and sequences in both real words and nonwords. Unlike the Semantic Feature Analysis (SFA) treatment—where training one word (e.g., "cat") can facilitate the retrieval of an untrained word (e.g., "mouse")—,the relationship between trained and untrained exemplars in PMT is less direct.

In PMT, word stimuli are selected based on two phonological sequence properties: (1) low phonotactic probability (the rarity of certain phonological sequences in a language); and (2) high phonological neighborhood density (the number of words differing by only one phoneme).

When PMT was first developed, the overall structure of phonological sequence knowledge was not well understood. The training and testing corpora were selected based on a hypothesis tested using a Parallel Distributed Processing (PDP) model. This model suggested that training atypical exemplars would improve the production of both typical and atypical exemplars, while training typical exemplars would benefit only typical ones. Atypical exemplars share features with typical ones, so training the former can enhance performance on both sets. In contrast, typical exemplars lack the distinctive features of atypical ones. The PDP model supported this hypothesis, and subsequent studies confirmed this effect, notably in semantic therapy for people with aphasia (Kiran & Thompson, 2003).

2.5   APPLICATIONS AND THERAPEUTIC APPROACHES

The description provided above suggests that therapeutic approaches for sound disorders may benefit from an informed understanding of phonological complexity. However, the field is still in its infancy, hindered by challenges such as the lack of a clear definition of syllabic complexity and limited linguistic training available to speech and language therapists worldwide.

Typically, assessments of phonological errors rely on simplistic measures like counting correct/incorrect sounds, failing to delve into the nuanced nature of these errors. Moreover, assessment batteries often present items incrementally from simple to complex, neglecting the *Complexity Account of Treatment Efficacy* (CATE; Thompson et al., 2003), which posits that training on complex structures can lead to generalization to less complex ones. Studies by Kiran and Thompson (2003) and Thompson and Shapiro (2007) support this notion CATE. For instance, Riley and Thompson (2015) explored the application of phonological complexity principles in training letter–sound correspondence reading for acquired phonological dyslexia. They found that training on more complex materials led to better generalization of untrained words compared to training on simpler materials.

In another study, Miozzo and Buchwald (2013) observed similar sonority effects in speech production for patients with phonological and phonetic sound production disorders, suggesting that sonority plays a role in both levels of processing. This finding indicates that sonority-based treatments could be effective for sound structure processing disorders, as they capture complexity at both phonological and phonetic levels.

2.6 Summary

Research into phonological and phonetic errors has highlighted a consistent trend: errors tend to decrease in relation to syllabic complexity, a phenomenon attributed to the sonority dispersion principle. This means that sounds are more likely to be omitted in contexts with complex onsets, as observed in various populations including individuals with aphasia, children, and second language learners.

Interestingly, both individuals with phonological difficulties and those with articulatory difficulties exhibit sensitivity to these syllabic constraints, suggesting universal sources of errors among people with aphasia. While the quantity of errors may vary between fluent and nonfluent speakers with aphasia, the underlying quality remains consistent.

Defining phonological complexity requires consideration beyond just syllable length or sound types; it also involves understanding preferences for simplified options. Future therapeutic protocols should incorporate measures of complexity that provide detailed explanations of error nature, drawing insights from the patient's spoken languages. This approach can offer a more nuanced understanding of errors and inform targeted interventions tailored to individual linguistic profiles.

2.7 Discussion Topics

1. Define syllabic complexity and the associated role of sonority, providing a couple of examples.
2. Discuss the sonority dispersion principles considering the syllabic simplification often reported in language acquisition. Present examples and implications for aphasic speech.
3. Present, with examples, some gradient of syllabic complexity, with examples from different kinds of aphasia.

4. Discuss how to map syllabic complexity in an intervention protocol, mentioning effects of syllabic complexity and items to be considered for generalizations.

5. Produce some possible phonological and phonetic errors that a patient with nonfluent aphasia could commit and explain the source of these errors. If you speak more than one language, please refer to all the languages you speak.

6. Considering the importance of coding phonological errors with linguistics informed systems, discuss the limit of the correct/incorrect coding system and how this could be modified.

REFERENCES

Clements, G. N. (1990). The role of the sonority cycle in core syllabification. In J. Kingston & M. Beckmann (Eds.), *Papers in laboratory phonology* (p. 1). Cambridge University Press.

Clements, G. N., & Keyser, S. J. (1983). *CV phonology: A generative theory of the syllable*. MIT Press.

Dell, G. S. (1986). A spreading activation theory of retrieval in sentence production. *Psychological Review, 93*, 283–321.

Dell, G. S. (1988). The retrieval of phonological forms in production: Tests and predictions from a connectionist model. *Journal of Memory and Language, 27*, 124–142.

Fromkin, V. (Ed.). (1973). *Speech errors as linguistic evidence*. Walter de Gruyter.

Goldrick, M., & Daland, R. (2009). Linking speech errors and phonological grammars: Insights from harmonic grammar networks. *Phonology, 26*(1), 147–185.

Greenberg, J. (1978). *Universals of human language. Vol 2: Phonology*. Stanford University Press.

Hume, E. (2003). Language specific markedness: The case of place of articulation. Studies in phonetics. *Phonology & Morphology, 9*(2), 295–310.

Ingram, D. (1974). Phonological rules in young children. *Journal of Child Language, 1*(1), 49–64.

Kaye, J., & Lowenstamm, J. (1981). Syllable structure and markedness theory. In A. Belletti, L. Brandi, & L. Rizzi (Eds.), *Theory of markedness in generative grammar* (pp. 287–315). Pacini Editore.

Kendall, D., & Nadeau, S. (2016). The phonomotor approach to treating phonological-based language deficits in people with aphasia. *Topics in Language Disorders, 36*(2), 109–122. https://doi.org/10.1097/TLD.000 0000000000085

Kiran, S., & Thompson, C. K. (2003). The role of semantic complexity in treatment of naming deficits: Training semantic categories in fluent aphasia by controlling exemplar typicality. *Journal of Speech, Language, and Hearing Research, 46*, 608–622.

Levelt, W. J. (1989). Working models of perception: Five general issues. In *Working models of perception* (pp. 489–503). Academic Press.

Levelt, W. J., Roelofs, A., & Meyer, A. S. (1999). A theory of lexical access in speech production. *Behavioral and Brain Sciences, 22*(1), 1–38.

Miozzo, M., & Buchwald, A. (2013). On the nature of sonority in spoken word production: Evidence from neuropsychology. *Cognition, 128*, 287–301. https://doi.org/10.1016/j.cognition.2013.04.006

Ohala, D. (1999). The influence of sonority on children's cluster reductions. *Journal of Communication Disorders, 32*, 397–422.

Paradis, C., & Beland, R. (2002). Syllabic constraints and constraints conflicts in loanword adaptations, aphasic speech and children's errors. In J. Durand & B. Laks (Eds.), *Phonetic, phonology and cognition* (pp. 191–225). Oxford University Press.

Riley, E. A., and Thompson, C. K. (2015). Training pseudoword reading in acquired dyslexia: A phonological complexity approach. *Aphasiology, 29*(2), 129–150.

Romani, C., & Calabrese, A. (1998). Syllabic constraints in the phonological errors of an aphasic patient. *Brain & Language, 64*, 83–121.

Romani, C., Olson, A., Semenza, C., & Grana', A. (2002). Patterns of phonological errors as a function of a phonological versus an articulatory locus of impairment. *Cortex, 38*, 541–567.

Smith, N. V. (1973). *The acquisition of phonology: A case study.* Cambridge University Press.

Spencer, A. (1988). Arguments for morpholexical rules1. *Journal of Linguistics, 24*(1), 1–29.

Stemberger, J. P. (1990). Wordshape errors in language production. *Cognition, 35*(2), 123–157.

Stemberger, J. P. (1991). Apparent anti-frequency effects in language production: The addition bias and phonological underspecification. *Journal of Memory and Language, 30*(2), 161–185.

Stemberger, J. P., & Bernhardt, B. H. (1997). Optimality theory. In *The new phonologies: Developments in clinical linguistics* (pp. 211–245).

Thompson, C. K., & Shapiro, L. P. (2007). Complexity in treatment of syntactic deficits. *American Journal of Speech-Language Pathology, 16*, 30–42.

Thompson, C. K., Shapiro, L. P., Kiran, S., & Sobecks, J. (2003). The role of syntactic complexity in treatment of sentence deficits in Agrammatic aphasia: The complexity account of treatment efficacy (CATE). *Journal of Speech, Language, and Hearing Research, 46*, 591–607.

CHAPTER 3

Disorders of Morphology in Aphasia

Abstract In this chapter we will review some stable findings on the impairment at the morphological level. Areas of difficulties for people with aphasia have been reported in the process of composition, where compound words are stored as the sum of their individual parts and the individual word that determines the word class of the compound is less affected than the other(s); in affixation, with a particular impairment in suffixation, the process that changes grammatical class in a word and – in some languages – contains syntactic information, over prefixation, which only changes word meaning; related to word classes, a dissociation between noun and verb production has been detected. Perhaps the most impaired part of morphology is arguably that on inflectional morphology on finite verbs, where a dissociation between verb tense and subject–verb agreement has been reported cross-linguistically and discussed extensively in the literature on aphasia.

Keywords Word class • Nouns vs. verbs • Grammatical classes • Compounds • Suffixes • Affixes • Prefixes • Derivation • Semantic feature analysis • Tense • Agreement

3.1   INTRODUCING MORPHOLOGY IN APHASIA

The morphological component of the language system is that which allows languages to create words and meanings from a set of words. Speakers can do so in many ways – for example, they can create a word with a different meaning and grammatical class by adding linguistic material to a **word stem** (from *create* to *creat-ive,* but also from *want* to *wanted*), or they can join words (stems) to create new words with a new meaning (from *ball* and *basket* to *basketball*). If you think of the way you speak, you will notice that you do this all the time. Most of the lexicon of a language is, in fact, *multimorphemic,* meaning it is made of words that can be divided into smaller units. Difficulties in this ability of combining units to make appropriate words can therefore be a great disadvantage for any speaker, and these have been extensively reported in patients with aphasia.

A productive operation in language is the conjunction of word stems to create novel words. This operation is called *composition.* In many languages, composition is a very creative mechanism, allowing not only same-grammatical class words to merge (i.e., noun – noun), but also words of different classes (i.e., verb – noun). German is one such example. The word *Kreuzfahrteilnehmer,* for example, is a composite word deriving from a noun verb (*teilnehmer*) and two nouns (*Kreuz* and *Fahr*), and it means "someone who takes part in a cruise trip." Typically, the compound word will have the same **features** as one of its elements, most frequently the rightmost. This element will give the compound its grammatical class (*overdose* is a noun, like *dose,* and not a preposition, like *over*) as well as other features like grammatical gender.

A different kind of word building is affixation. Affixes are linguistic material which is added to word stems. The addition can be at the front of the word (*prefixation*), at the end of the word (*suffixation*), or, more rarely, in between (*infixation*). Affixes can be either *derivational* or *inflectional.* Derivational affixation modifies word meaning (*school > pre-school*) and sometimes its class (swift $_{ADJECTIVE}$ > Swiftly $_{ADVERB}$). Inflectional affixes do not modify the class or meaning of the stem, but they do add information. Inflection on nouns expresses the features of that noun, namely number (singular/plural), and grammatical gender (masculine/feminine/neutral). Different languages behave differently in terms of both where they admit inflectional morphology, and which type they employ. English, for instance, has overt number inflectional morphology on nouns but not adjectives, and no gender morphology. Italian, on the other hand, expresses both number and gender on all elements of the noun phrase in 1: the noun *occh-i* (eyes) contains the masculine plural inflection -i. This is reflected in the article (i, the, plural), the possessive adjective (*suo-i,* his/her, plural) and the adjective (*azzurr-i,* blue, plural).

(1) I suoi occhi azzurri 'His/her blue eyes'

On the verb, inflectional morphology identifies information such as the time and mood of the action. In 2, *was* is inflected for past tense, and *going* for a progressive state. As you can see, verbal inflectional morphology is crucial to provide the correct decription of the action.

(2) He *was* go-*ing* to the supermarket.

In this chapter, we are focusing on disfunctions in composition and inflection which have been consistently reported for people with aphasia.

3.2   Composition in Aphasia

As complex, multimorphemic entities, compounds such as the English *blueberry* or the Italian *febbre gialla* can be hard to process, use, and repeat. In recent years, a substantial amount of studies on acquired language impairments have investigated the behaviour of a disrupted language system on morphologically complex words. Evidence of impaired production of compounds, with accuracy often as low as chance level, has been reported (Blanken, 2000). Crucially, the responses given by people with aphasia show that the compound is accessed either wholly (leading to a correct answer) or partially. Partial access is either access to one of the components of the word, a process known as *simplification,* or access to the semantics of the word, but not its morphology. The latter type of error is evident when people with aphasia provide a periphrasis of the compounds (*semantic paraphasia*). Examples from German are provided below:

(3) Target: Papierkorb (wastepaper basket).
   Semantic paraphasia: Papier zu wegwerfen, *to throw away paper.*
   Simplification: Korb, *basket.*

Results in this direction from impaired speakers have been crucial to provide evidence for the mechanism of morphological decomposition in lexical processing, namely the process of decomposing a word into its constituent morphemes. Several models have been proposed to account for the role of morphological information in complex word processing, which propose different stages in which morphological information comes into play in word processing, and different units of morphological decomposition (see Stevens & Plaut, 2022 for a recent overview).

Of particular interest in this sense is the error of *simplification.* This has been suggested to be influenced by the characteristics of the components, namely their order and their frequency. Low frequency-first compounds, in fact, are understood to be harder to access than high frequency-first compounds. Crucially, people with aphasia show sensitivity to these characteristics. In languages like English and German, where the rightmost word in the compound is the one providing the whole compound its grammatical features, its omission would result in an omission of the grammatical features of the compound. In people with aphasia, the most omitted of the two (or more) components is usually one(s) that is *not* responsible for the grammatical class of the compound. This was demonstrated, for example, in a study on bilingual aphasic speakers (Semenza & Mondini, 2015). In the study, two languages with different preferences on the position of the element in compounds determining grammatical class: were tested: English, where this is usually the rightmost element; and French, where it can be both the rightmost and the leftmost element. Consequently, all French stimuli created for the experiment were left-element-dominant, and all English stimuli were right-element-dominant. Results from reading, repeating, and translating compounds revealed that French-English bilingual patients showed a left-constituent advantage in accuracy for the French stimuli, and a right-constituent advantage in English, confirming that they were sensitive to the centrality of each component in determining the features of the compound.

3.3   Affixation in Aphasia

The impairment that has received the most attention for aphasia, particularly due to its implication for linguistic theory, is that of affixation and, more specifically, of inflection. More specifically, an asymmetry has been detected in acquired language disorders between *derivational* and *inflectional* morphology, with inflection being more severely compromised than derivation inflection. This asymmetry was first described by Miceli and Caramazza (1988), who explored the production of both derivational and inflectional morphology in an aphasic speaker of Italian in a comprehensive assessment featuring word repetition and spontaneous speech. This speaker produced a nonnegligible number of morphological errors such as affix omission in all derived words (prefixed and suffixed). In a task specifically investigating the repetition of prefixed words, which contained both actual prefixed words (*"dis-grazia,"* disgrace) and pseudoprefixed words (*"discorso,"* speech), the speaker was below chance in the correct repetition of the stimuli. However, when distinguished between suffixed and prefixed words, most errors were found to be in suffixes, which contain inflectional information in Italian, and not in prefixes, which are derivational affixes in Italian. Prefixation has been generally described as showing great individual variation, as shown in studies where some participants present a selective disadvantage for prefixed over non-prefixed words, while others do not (Semenza et al., 2002; Ciaccio et al., 2020). For models of morphological decomposition, this profile of impaired derivational morphology is evidence of the fact that derived words are accessed as stems + affixes. The most common types of errors in aphasic speakers (omissions, substitutions) show that the processing of affixes may be hard, but there is still strong awareness of the function of affixes and their place in word formation.

Crucially, an asymmetry between derivational and inflectional morphology signals an impairment at the level of morphosyntactic operations, rather than just of word formation. Otherwise, all affixes would be treated similarly.

Not just aphasia. As we will discuss in Chap. 7, some of the impairments of language that are reported within this book are not limited to aphasia. A number of the impairments in morphology under discussion in this chapter are reported across language disorders. At the level of derivational morphology, for example, impairments in the production of affixes that determine a word class change are reported in both neurodevelopmental and degenerative disorders. Dyslexia is a neurodevelopmental learning disorder which is characterized by difficulties with accurate and/or fluent word decoding. Speakers with dyslexia have been shown to have difficulties in reading suffixed words. Crucially, they are worse at reading real suffixed words (louder) than on pseudosuffixed words (baker), confirming that the difficulty lies in the morphological process of affixation (Rastle et al., 2006). Dementia is a degenerative condition with several possible causes, most prominently abnormal neuronal cell death. Some patients with dementia have been shown to have poorer performance than healthy controls in producing derived nouns (Auclair-Ouellet et al., 2017). Crucially, asymmetries in the hardest derivational processes are reported in dementia and aphasia. Testing agreement and tense marking in Greek people with dementia and possible Alzheimer's disease (a specific type of dementia), Fyndanis et al. (2013) find that participants perform overall worse than controls in production of correct morphology. The authors also find that, for most of their participants, tense morphology was harder than agreement morphology, like people with aphasia.

Strong cross-linguistic evidence collected in recent decades has pointed to even more selective impairment in inflectional morphology, namely one on tense inflection on verbs as opposed to agreement inflection on verbs and nouns/adjectives. This dissociation has, in turn, given rise to several theoretical approaches to the morphological impairment in aphasia. In one of the most influential early papers exploring verbal inflectional morphology in aphasia, Friedmann and Grodzinsky (1997) explore sentence completion, sentence repetition, and spontaneous productions of an aphasic speaker of Hebrew, a language with rich and easily distinguishable inflectional morphology. Verbs are overtly inflected both for time (3 possible tenses) and for agreement (10 agreement forms), and each inflectional operation is expressed on a different morpheme, which allows for a clear dissociation between errors on the operation of tense inflection agreement (remove agreement) and gender/number/person agreement. Strikingly, the authors find a clear dissociation between agreement, which was intact, and tense inflection, which was prone to error in their participant. For instance, in the oral sentence completion task, which is exemplified in 4 below, the participant only made 1 agreement error, whereas she made errors of tense agreement inflection (remove agreement) in exactly 50% of conditions. Of these, 70% were errors on a copula and 38% on a lexical verb.

(4) Yesterday the boy walked.
4a. Tense condition: Tomorrow the boy _____ (walk, future)
4b. Agreement condition: Yesterday the boys _____ (walk, past, plural).

Because all are instances of inflectional morphology, it must be the case that something is differentiating them that is not strictly at the level of morphology, but rather at the interface with syntax. This pattern has led to the postulation of a series of theoretical accounts of the hierarchy of these features on the syntactic tree (for example the Tree Pruning Hypothesis, TPH, Friedmann and Grodzinsky, 1997) and the distinction between types of features (like in the Tense Underspecification Hypothesis, TUH, Wenzlaff & Clahsen 2004, 2005) and different postulations on the existence of a specific locus of impairment in aphasic speakers.

3.4   Assessments of Morphology

Not many assessments exist for aphasia that are targeted to morphology. The Northwestern Assessment of Verb Inflection (NAVI) was designed to examine the production of verb inflection forms in individuals with language disorders resulting from neurological disease. The NAVI is used to assess one's ability to produce finite (present singular, present plural, past regular and irregular forms) and nonfinite (infinitive, present progressive) verb inflection forms in English, using a sentence completion task (Lee & Thompson, 2017).

3.5   Applications and Therapeutic Approaches

Given its prominence for sentence formation as well as intelligibility, verb inflection is the area of morpho(syntax) that is mostly assessed in treatment. A meta-analysis on single-case studies of verb treatments by De Aguiar et al. (2016) showed that verb inflection treatments are effective in generalizing tense production to untreated verbs at sentence level. One of the most successful treatments of this kind is ACTION (Bastiaanse et al., 1997).

Two studies report on the treatment of verbal morphology by means of a Computerized Visual Communication protocol (C-VIC, Weinrich et al., 1997, 1999). C-VIC utilizes a set of pictures or icons in a hierarchical database. Icons represent people, objects, actions, prepositional relationships, and quantification. Patients navigate through the computerized tsk and are encouraged to verbalize what they see. Corrected responses are provided by the therapist. This treatment was used to elicit past, present, and future tense forms of regular and irregular verbs in sentences. In both studies, the production of inflected verbs in sentences improved, and generalization was observed in the use of morphological transformations, but not in verb retrieval.

Originally developed in Dutch, it was later adapted to German (Bastiaanse et al., 2006) and Italian (de Aguiar et al., 2015). In ACTION, verb inflection is trained in different forms and in different positions in the sentence following four steps, as in Table 3.1:

This method was proven effective in generalizing correct verb inflection from trained to untrained verbs (Bastiaanse et al., 2006).

Table 3.1   Steps for the ACTION training (adapted from Bastiaanse et al., 2006)

Step 1	Action naming	This is a preparatory step in which verb retrieval at word level is trained by action naming in response to pictures.
Step 2	Retrieval of infinitive in sentence context	The participant sees a picture and reads a sentence in which the verb in the infinitival form is left out. The participant is instructed to fill in the missing verb orally.
Step 3	Retrieval of finite verb in sentence context	The participant sees a picture and reads a sentence in which the verb in finite form is left out. The participant is instructed to fill in the missing verb orally.
Step 4	Sentence construction with finite verbs	The participant sees a picture and is instructed to construct a sentence to describe it.

3.6   SUMMARY

In this chapter, we explored some of the characterizing aspects of one of the most reported difficulties in aphasia, namely that of morphology. Within word boundaries, we saw that word building is also problematic in the presence of an impairment of naming, and that the impairment is often systematic, mostly affecting the part of the word that is less crucial in determining the features of the final word in compounds, and the part of the word that does not change the grammatical class of the word in affixed words. While derivational morphology is mostly spared, we highlighted, on the other hand, that inflectional morphology has been robustly found to be more impaired in this population across the board, and, in languages with rich morphology, within inflectional morphology, tense to be more impaired than agreement operations. This may be due to syntax being more preserved than morphology, leading to morphological elements with heavier weight in the syntactic makeup of the sentence being retained more than others.

3.7   DISCUSSION TOPICS

1. Discuss the processes involved in building compounds and provide examples from your mother tongue, identifying potential areas of difficulty for aphasic speakers. For example, do you think compound words in your language would be mostly affected in their leftward or rightward element?
2. Prefixes and suffixes behave differently in aphasia. Discuss why that is (hint: most suffixes are classified as inflectional morphology).
3. Grammatical class is crucial in determining the degree of the impairment in word naming. Discuss what this implies providing examples.
4. Look at definitions of composition, derivation and inflection in Sect. 3.1 and provide other examples. Reflect on the derivation and its relationship with word category.
5. Provide examples of possible errors that can occur in bilingual aphasia and if they occur due to attrition between languages or a genuine lack of competence due to aphasia.

REFERENCES

Auclair-Ouellet, N., Fossard, M., Laforce, R., Jr., Bier, N., & Macoir, J. (2017). Conception or *conceivation? The processing of derivational morphology in semantic dementia. *Aphasiology, 31*(2), 166–188.

Bastiaanse, R., Hurkmans, J., & Links, P. (2006). The training of verb production in Broca's aphasia: A multiple-baseline across-behaviours study. *Aphasiology, 20*, 298–311. https://doi.org/10.1080/02687030500474922

Bastiaanse, R., Jonkers, R., Quak, C. H., & Varela Put, M. (1997). *Werkwoordproductie op Woord en Zinsniveau [Verb production at the word and sentence level]*. Swets Test Publishers.

Blanken, G. (2000). The production of nominal compounds in aphasia. *Brain and Language, 74*, 84–102.

Ciaccio, L. A., Burchert, F., & Semenza, C. (2020). Derivational morphology in Agrammatic aphasia: A comparison between prefixed and suffixed words. *Frontiers in Psychology, 11*, 1070. https://doi.org/10.3389/fpsyg.2020.01070

de Aguiar, V., Bastiaanse, R., Capasso, R., Gandolfi, M., Smania, N., Rossi, G., & Miceli, G. (2015). Can tDCS enhance item-specific effects and generalization after linguistically motivated aphasia therapy for verbs? *Frontiers in Behavioral Neuroscience, 9*, 190.

De Aguiar, V., Bastiaanse, R., & Miceli, G. (2016). Improving production of treated and untreated verbs in aphasia: A meta-analysis. *Frontiers in Human Neuroscience, 10*, 468.

Friedmann, N., & Grodzinsky, Y. (1997). Tense and agreement in agrammatic production: Pruning the syntactic tree. *Brain and Language, 56*, 397–425.

Fyndanis, V., Manouilidou, C., Koufou, E., Karampekios, S., & Tsapakis, E. M. (2013). Agrammatic patterns in Alzheimer's disease: Evidence from tense, agreement, and aspect. *Aphasiology, 27*, 178–200. https://doi.org/10.1080/0268703 8.2012.705814

Lee, J., & Thompson, C. K. (2017). Northwestern assessment of verb inflection. Evanston, IL: Northwestern University.

Miceli, G., & Caramazza, A. (1988). Dissociation of inflectional and derivational morphology. *Brain and Language, 35*, 24–65. https://doi.org/10.1016/0093-934X(88)90100-9

Rastle, K., Tyler, L. K., & Marslen-Wilson, W. (2006). New evidence for morphological errors in deep dyslexia. *Brain and Language, 97*(2), 189–199. https://doi.org/10.1016/j.bandl.2005.10.003

Semenza, C., & Mondini, S. (2015). Word-formation in aphasia. In P. O. Müller, I. Ohnheiser, S. Olsen, & F. Rainer (Eds.), *Word-formation: An international handbook of the languages of Europe* (pp. 2154–2177). De Gruyter Mouton.

Semenza, G., Girelli, L., Spacal, M., Kobal, J., & Mesec, A. (2002). Derivation by prefixation: Two aphasia case studies. *Brain and Language, 81*, 242–249.

Stevens, P., & Plaut, D. C. (2022). From decomposition to distributed theories of morphological processing in reading. *Psychonomic Bulletin & Review, 29*(5), 1673–1702.

Weinrich, M., Boser, K. I., & McCall, D. (1999). Representation of linguistic rules in the brain: Evidence from training an aphasic patient to produce past tense verb morphology. *Brain and Language, 70*, 144–158. https://doi.org/10.1006/brln.1999.2141

Weinrich, M., Shelton, J. R., Cox, D. M., & McCall, D. (1997). Remediating production of tense morphology improves verb retrieval in chronic aphasia. *Brain and Language, 58*, 23–45. https://doi.org/10.1006/brln.1997.1757

Wenzlaff, M., & Clahsen, H. (2004). Tense and agreement in German agrammatism. *Brain and Language, 89*(1), 57–68. https://doi.org/10.1016/S0093-934X(03)00298-0

Wenzlaff, M., & Clahsen, H. (2005). Finiteness and verb-second in German agrammatism. *Brain and Language, 92*(1), 33–44. https://doi.org/10.1016/j.bandl.2004.05.006

CHAPTER 4

Disorders of Semantics in Aphasia

Abstract Many people with aphasia have difficulty in determining the relationship between words and their meaning. Word naming, namely the ability to name objects, is severely affected in aphasia (something which is often described as word retrieval deficit). The semantic features of the words have been shown to have an impact on how easily these can be retrieved in aphasia. Pronoun resolution, namely the ability to properly utilize reference to the nouns that need to be interpreted in relation to the previous context, is another area of difficulty for patients with aphasia (PWA). PWA often struggle to correctly identify the referent of pronouns. In this chapter we will look at the semantic aspects that are at the source of the deficit and forms of treatments proposed to overarch the impairment.

Keywords Reference • Deixis • Anaphora resolution • Pronouns • Animacy • Imageability • Word retrieval • Semantic traits • Gesture treatments

4.1 Introducing Semantics in Aphasia

The definition 'semantic aphasia' describes an impairment in semantic processing, principally regarding the set of abilities that allow individuals to access and manipulate linguistic context, namely word and sentence meanings, and their relation to the extralinguistic context within which

© The Author(s), under exclusive license to Springer Nature Switzerland AG 2024
M. Garraffa, G. Smith, *Linguistic Theory for Aphasia*,
https://doi.org/10.1007/978-3-031-77134-7_4

they are pronounced. One of the first pieces of information about a language we must interpret, once we have decoded sounds, is the meaning of individual words in their context. Firstly, we must decode what *type* of word it is i.e., we must establish its **word class.** The main meaningful distinction between word classes is between words that contain semantic information on an object or action (**content words,** like *lottery, grand-dad, recycle*) and those which only serve a grammatical purpose (**function words,** like *the, an, with, that*).

In semantics, word meaning (of content words) is theorized as the expression of a list of finite fundamental traits that describe the nature of all things of the world, called **semantic traits or semantic features.** These semantic traits are typically binary categories of features that each entity either possesses (visualized as +) or does not (visualized as –). For instance, the word *boy* expresses a meaning which possesses values for traits of being animate, human, male, and young (+human, +animate, +male, –old). To further understand the meaning of the words we encounter with respects to the extralinguistic context, we must interpret the connection between words of a natural language, referred to in semantics as *signifiers*, and the entity of the physical world they are referring to, sometimes called a *signified*, or *discourse referent*. One example of a signified is the four-wheeled means of transportation we may use to go to work, and the signifier for such entity is the word *car* in the English language, *voiture* in French, and so on. The relation between a signifier and a linguistic element indicating it is not 1:1. In fact, the same referent can be identified in language using different linguistic elements, as shown in the examples in (1). Both *a cat* and *it* refer to the same element of the outside world in this context.

(1)   *A cat* crossed the road. Hannah gave *it* food.

Among the linguistic expressions we can use to refer to something, nouns (such as *A cat* in 1) explicitly denote the identity of the discourse referent. On the other hand, pronouns (*it*) share some semantic and grammatical features with the discourse referent. For the discourse referent to be correctly identified, a relation between the pronoun and the referent must be established.

Aphasic word retrieval and bilingualism. We have mentioned that word retrieval can be affected in aphasia, although this can be specific to selected categories of words. But what happens when the speaker is bilingual? Bilingualism is shown to improve nonverbal cognitive abilities, but at the same time it makes language processing more effortful, particularly in tasks such as word retrieval, when it is claimed that the language that is not being activated needs to be suppressed (see Bialystok et al., 2009 for a comprehensive review). The study of bilingualism in aphasia has gained considerable momentum. Some studies exploring word retrieval in bilingual aphasics confirm that it is generally impaired in bilingual speakers too. In a case study on a multilingual fluent anomic aphasic speaker with dominant Greek and non-dominant English, Kambanaros (2016) tested written and oral word naming in both languages. Results reveal that the participant was equally impaired in word naming across most conditions, thus revealing neither a facilitatory nor an inhibitory role of bilingualism. Interestingly, a dissociation only appeared in writing to dictation, where Greek (the home language and the language of literacy) was more preserved.

Looking at semantics more specifically, some studies are interested in investigating to what extent semantic processing is shared between the two languages in bilinguals, with some studies concurring that bilinguals show a similar activation when they are processing words from L1 or L2. In a study on semantic control during the speech production of aphasic bilinguals, Calabria et al. (2019) test 11 Catalan–Spanish aphasic bilinguals and a group of controls on a semantic blocked cycling naming task. In this task, participants were required to name semantically related or semantically unrelated blocks of pictures. General language measures showed that only one of the eleven patients showed an imbalanced impairment towards their non-dominant language, while all others showed parallel language deficits. Overall, semantic interference (the related vs unrelated factor) was greater in patients with aphasia than in controls and, most importantly here, it was greater in their non-dominant language, despite the apparent parallel language deficit.

Semantic aphasia is characterized as a difficulty in any task requiring access to meaning. This impairment is described as the consequence of limited access to the internal storage of meaning and representations (see Mirman & Britt, 2014), and is thereofre considered to be tightly linked to non-linguistic cognitive abilities such as working memory, inhibition and control (Tessaro et al., 2022).

4.2   Lexical Retrieval

One of the most evident and frequent areas of difficulty identified in PWA is in word naming. The resulting impairment is usually described as *anomia* (from *a* indicating absence and *nomen*, name). The ability to name words, more specifically called *lexical retrieval*, refers to the access and selection of a target **lemma** at the specific time when this is needed. Lexical retrieval is understood to be a composite phenomenon made of different stages, from access to the semantic value of a word (i.e., its meaning) to access to its phonological output (i.e., how it is pronounced), and so on. Anomia can result in hesitations, rephrasing or paraphrasing, tip-of-the-tongue phenomena (namely zero responses, typically accompanied by a feeling of frustration), or in the substitution of the word with other, irrelevant words, or even with made-up words (the latter case is referred to as *paraphasia*). Impairments in lexical retrieval in PWA have been found to arise from different causes, namely the loci of the impairment can be at any stage of the process of retrieval (see Nickels, 2001 for a comprehensive discussion). For example, impairments can appear at the level of semantic specifications, of the access to the phonological output lexicon of the words, and so on.

A similar case can be made for a dissociation in word naming. Specifically, it has been proposed that anomic speakers find lexical retrieval particularly challenging overall, but have no or limited difficulties with retrieving verb information. On the other hand, agrammatic speakers manifest a more severe difficulty in the retrieval of verbs over retrieval of nouns in lexical retrieval tasks. In neuropsychology, this dissociation and its relation to different lesions has been taken to be an indicator that some parts of the brain are sensitive to the different grammatical categories (Damasio & Tranel, 1993; Shapiro & Caramazza, 2003a, 2003b). Importantly, it has been suggested that this asymmetry is not generalized to all PWA with difficulties in lexical retrieval; rather, it is more evident in those PWA who show impaired syntax (sometimes referred to as *agrammatics*, as we will see in Chap. 5) (Miceli et al., 1984; Luzzatti et al., 2006). Luzzatti et al.

(2006) tested lexical retrieval via a visual naming task with objects and actions and showed that the overall performance of PWA was worse than that of controls in naming, with no dissociation between verbs and nouns. However, when looking at the pattern of fluent and non-fluent speakers in the PWA group, a difference between nouns and verbs emerged in nonfluent PWA. A greater dissociation between nouns and verbs with respects to controls in non-fluent PWA with respect to fluent speakers was also observed in spontaneous speech (Crepaldi et al., 2011). Like controls, fluent PWA showed a high rate of verb and noun productions in their speech. Conversely, nonfluent PWA showed overall lower counts and noun/verb asymmetry, producing lower number of verb types than fluent PWA and controls. Importantly, the difference emerges at the level of *tokens*, namely the number of different productions of the same stems, with the verb-specific impairment emerging in nonfluent patients only as an inferior production of different inflected verb forms. This suggests a difficulty at the level of production of verb morphology. Some features have been proposed to negatively affect word retrieval in some PWA. For instance, semantic features, including animacy and imageability, have been shown to influence noun retrieval (see Luzzatti et al., 2006 and references therein). In verb naming, grammatical characteristics such as the complexity of the argument structure have been shown to influence performance in verb production (Thompson et al., 1997).

Another phenomenon that has been discussed for anomic aphasia is that of semantic **category-specific deficits**. Patients with category-specific semantic deficits show asymmetric impairments for one semantic category compared to other semantic categories. In Fig. 4.1 (Mahon & Caramazza, 2009), we can see some interesting examples of asymmetric lexical retrieval patterns in PWA. Figure 4.1a shows an asymmetry in two patients between animate and inanimate objects (dog vs. car), which we shall be discussing in the next section, but other curious distinctions exist, such as that between fruits and vegetables and non-living things (pear vs. pan). Here, we will be looking at some of the arguably most relevant semantic traits. A review can be found in Nickels et al. (2022).

Animacy. Animacy is the extent to which a word/concept possesses the property of being alive and/or sentient. [+animate] is typically associated with living things of the world such as humans and animals; [−animate] is associated with objects or abstract concepts, such as "time" or "sugar." This semantic feature is shown to be a predictor of accuracy in people with aphasia steadily across the literature. In a case report of a

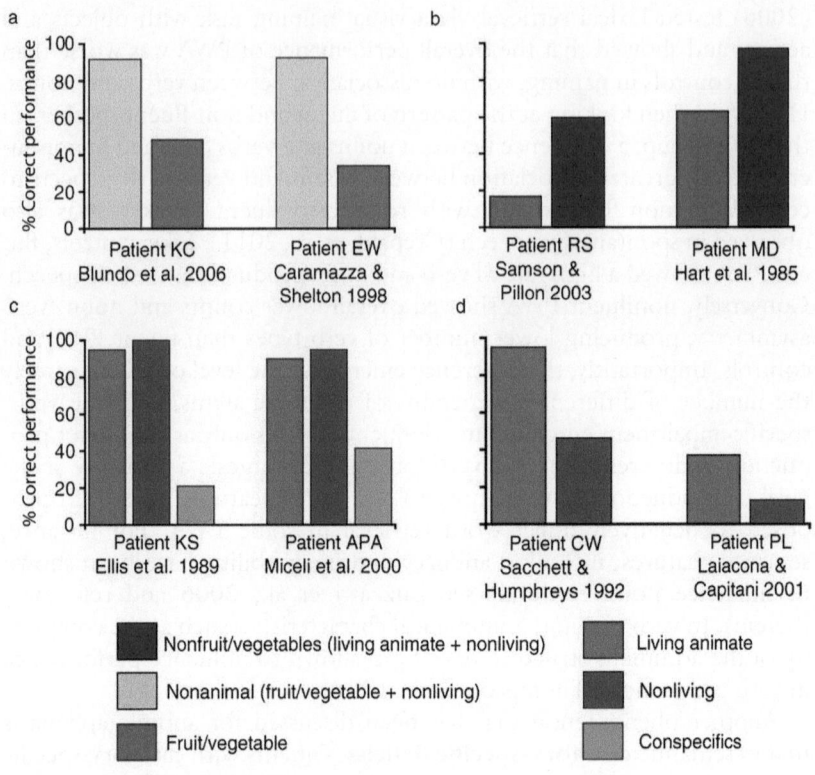

Mahon BZ, Caramazza A. 2009.
Annu. Rev. Psychol. 60:27–51

Fig. 4.1 Picture-naming performance across different semantic traits: (a) living animate vs nonanimal; fruits and vegetables vs non-fruit/vegetables; conspecifics (belonging to the same species) vs non-conspecifics animate and inanimate; living animate vs non-living. Image by Mahon and Caramazza (2009)

Mandarin Chinese-speaking anomic patient, for instance, Bi et al. (2007) employ a picture-naming task with animate and inanimate items that were matched on frequency, familiarity, word length, and imageability, and find animacy to be a main predictor of accuracy in one patient. Similar results were achieved in Laiacona and Capitani with an Italian speaker (2001).

Concreteness and countability. 'Concreteness effect' is the advantage for the retrieval of concrete over abstract words robustly reported across tasks in semantic aphasia (e.g., Franklin et al., 1995 for lexical retrieval. See Paivio, 1991 for a review). Semantic aphasics generally show an advantage in retrieving words such as *table*, which is –animate, + concrete, over words such as *peace*, which is –animate, –concrete. Interestingly, the reverse pattern, or 'reverse concreteness effect', has been reported mostly in semantic dementia in the form of a selective impairment in concrete nouns, which might be the result of a brain decay in areas which are deemed to be related to abstract representations (e.g., Papagno et al., 2009).

Countability. [–countable] nouns (or **mass nouns**) represent substances or aggregates, such as water or flour; they are semantically plurals and are treated as an undifferentiated unit, rather than as something with discrete elements. [+countable] nouns (or **count nouns**) represent objects with clear boundaries, such as people and animals; they can be modified by quantity and occur in both singular and plural forms. Similarly to concreteness, countability can also affect semantic aphasia. In Herbert and Best (2010), the authors use a picture-naming task with bare countable and uncountable nouns ("This is _," i.e., "This is bread") and one with the determiner a/an for countable nouns and some for uncountable nouns ("This is a /some _," i.e., "This is a ball," "This is some flour"). Overall, the participant showed an asymmetry whereby naming count nouns was easier than naming uncountable nouns. Most of the participant's errors were omissions or substitutions of the mass count noun determiner with the singular count noun determiner "a/an" (e.g. "This is a water").

4.3   Pronoun Resolution

Establishing a relationship between a discourse referent and its external referent is a crucial ability to understand the meaning of sentences. To be correctly interpreted and used, deictics -namely all those elements that take a different referent depending on the time and place they are used- need to be linked to linguistic (or extralinguistic) material which precedes them in the discourse. In aphasia, as well as in other atypical speakers, several studies have reported difficulties in this operation for pronouns. This may result in overuse or underuse of pronouns. When pronouns are overused, they are used even when too little information is given to interpret their reference; when they are underused there is an overreliance on lexical elements, even when pronouns would be preferred in that context (Gleason et al., 1980; Ulatowska et al., 1983).

For comprehension, Chapman and Ulatowska (1989) designed tell–retell stories where they manipulated whether the referents following two nouns were nouns or pronouns and tested aphasic patients and healthy controls in their accuracy in the identification of the elements that referred to the same entity (an ability called **reference resolution**). Participants heard a story and were instructed to repeat it in their own words; they were also asked to identify the participants of each sentence. Examples of the story are given in (2a) and (2b). As the gender of the pronoun can be a linguistic facilitator in pronoun resolution, participants were shown cards with the image of the customer and the waitress, showing that both were female.

(2a) Pronoun version: The customer shouted angrily at the waitress that the meal was awful. She was new at the job and did not know how to respond. She hoped the food would be better next time. She was still mad and threw the food at the chef.

(2b) Noun version: The customer shouted angrily at the waitress that the meal was awful. The waitress was new at the job and did not know how to respond. The waitress hoped the food would be better next time. The customer was still mad and threw the food at the chef.

(from Chapman & Ulatowska, 1989)

While controls did not show difficulties with identifying referents in either condition, aphasic subjects showed an impairment, which was significantly higher in the condition with pronouns in (2a). Interpreting pronouns, which are not highly descriptive about a specific referent, may be harder given the absence of semantic cues provided by the lexical element which, in this case, give an indication of the roles (customers are more plausibly angry about food, and waitresses are more plausibly new at the job). For production, underuse of pronouns and, more generally, of deitics, was reported in Parsons (1993).

Parsons (1993) explored the use of single anaphoric expressions in aphasia testing use of the four major types of deixis categories in a discourse task and an elicitation task, as exemplified in (3).

(3) i. **PERSON DEIXIS**: A. Speaker – first person B. Addressee – second person C. Kinship terms D. Assumed role – first person E. Assumed role – second person

ii. **PLACE DEIXIS**: A. Identifying: THIS, THAT B. Informing-I: HERE, THERE C. Informing-II: RIGHT, LEFT, UP, DOWN

     D. Acknowledging I – verbs of motion: COME, BRING
     E. Acknowledging II – verbs of motion: GO, TAKE
  iii. **TIME DEIXIS**: A. Now B. Immediately following now C. Immediately preceding now D. Immediately following now +1 E. Immediately preceding now −1
  iv. **SOCIAL DEIXIS**: A. Familiar B. Polite C. Titles D. Mr. and Mrs. E. Sir/Ma'am

(adapted from Parsons, 1993)

Overall, participants with non-fluent aphasia were found to produce fewer deictics than their healthy counterparts. Aphasic speakers produced more non-deictic responses in the elicitation task compared to controls, producing a lexical noun phrase in place of the anaphoric element. Lexical responses increased with the level of severity of aphasia, as did the use of gestures, a non-linguistic type of deixis, in place of linguistic deixis.

On the other hand, an example of overuse comes from corpus data from Spanish speakers. Martínez-Ferreiro et al. (2019) explored the number of occurrences and diversity of forms of different types of connectors and pronouns. In general, PWA were found to overuse the subject pronouns, more so in the case of the non-fluent than the fluent patients, as exemplified in (4). Because subject pronouns are not necessary in most environments in Spanish, where subject pronouns are generally omitted unless it serves a specific purpose (such as **focus**), overuse is a semantic violation, violating principles of accessibility theory, namely giving too much information on an already accessible referent.

(4) (yo) Quiero verlo
(I)Want-to see-it.
'I want to see it'.

4.4   Semantic Properties of the Copula

As we have discussed in Chap. 3, verb morphology is a known area of disadvantage in aphasia. This impairment often shows a disadvantage on tense morphology over agreement morphology, and it has been replicated across languages. As we will discuss here, tense morphology on verbs is not easy to test in English speakers as the verbal morphology in English just inflects for past tense (-ed) and present progressive (-ing), but the semantic properties of the copula are crucial to investigate this impairment in English speakers. This is a good example of how information from linguistic theoretical frameworks may be crucial in improving patient assessment (i.e., for English tense impairment).

Arabatzi and Edwards' (2002) study of English agrammatic patients illustrated both the replacement and the omission of verbal inflections through task-elicited and spontaneous language. In a typical narrative task, participants are shown a series of images depicting a story and are asked to retell it in their own words. In a sentence completion task, the authors elicited the use of inflected verbs by providing the context for a past tense, for example by showing a picture of a girl drawing a house and asking participants to read and complete (5).

(5) She is drawing a house. Yesterday she ___ a rose.

Omission errors were of the type exemplified in (6), namely bare stem productions (6a) and auxiliary omission in progressive tenses (6b).

(6a) Yesterday she draw (target: drew) a house.
(6b) Tomorrow she cook (target: will cook) a cake.

While errors of verb morphology have been detected, a fine-grained analysis of the morphological impairment in tense like the ones we have discussed in (3) has not been possible so far given the nature of the English inflectional system, which is morphologically poor. Smith et al. (2023) recently proposed a framework that taps into semantics to explore deficits in the verbal domain in English by investigating the verb *to be*, a very frequent verbal form.

Following Carlson (1977), copula (the verb *to be*) can be used in two different predications: in individual-level (IL) predicates, which denote fundamental, integral features of the referent (7a); and in stage-level (SL) predicates, which denote temporal or geographical impermanence that are subject to a specific event (7b).

(7a) Bob is a frog (IL)
(7b) Bob is in the castle (SL)

Both predicates are expressed with the same morphological word (is), but their semantics are different. Building on a framework initially proposed for child language (Becker, 2002, 2004) where SL predicates are acquired later compared to IL, Smith et al. (2023) analyzed the production of copula in a group of PWA. They found a higher rate of copula omission in SL predicates compared to IL, with PWA producing sentences like the one in (8).

(8) "but still, something missing" (patient BU07a)

Analyzing the spontaneous speech of 16 aphasic patients, the authors find SL predicates to be the primary site of *to be* omission, with the implication that the verb *to be* can be a productive tool to investigate if the temporal information on the verb necessary in SL predicates is impaired. The results supported an impairment of Tense as well as a dissociation between tense inflection and agreement; incorrect agreement was scarce across all participants while impaired tense inflection was observed both through copula deletions and flawed subject Case assignment. This pattern is convergent with that of the adopted framework (Becker, 2002, 2004), therefore providing further support with data from aphasia that a fragile tense inflection results in a selective vulnerability of copulas of SL predicates.

4.5   ASSESSMENT OF SEMANTICS IN APHASIA

The most common tasks to assess semantic processing in patients with neurological conditions rely on verbal processing capacities. Tasks that target verbal processing include confrontation naming and category fluency for production and spoken word to picture matching for comprehension. Tasks of this kind are included in several comprehensive diagnostic tools, but very few adequately examine both the production and the comprehension of nouns and verbs. This is the case, for example, for the Western Aphasia Battery-Revised (WAB, Kertesz, 2007). The WAB-R was indicated as a test of choice in the international Research Outcome Measuring Aphasia (ROMA) study (Wallace et al., 2019), and it has been adapted into several languages, including Korean (Kim & Na, 2004) and Bangla (Keshree et al., 2013). The observed language behaviors classify the patient as having a specific type of aphasia, including anomia thanks to a section on lexical processing which includes object naming and verbal fluency. Similar measures are contained in the Boston Naming Test (BNT; Kaplan et al., 1983), the Boston Diagnostic Aphasia Examination (BDAE; Goodglass et al., 2001) and the Psycholinguistic Assessment of Language Processing in Aphasia (PALPA; Kay et al., 1996). In contrast, other tools evaluate verb production and comprehension, for example the Verb and Sentence Test (VAST; Bastiaanse et al., 2003). These will be discussed in the next chapter on syntax. A recent tool that aims at assessing the comprehension and production of names and verbs is the Northwestern Naming Battery (Thompson et al., 2016), which elicits the naming of object and verbs in different syntactic contexts.

Another recent and still relatively unexplored area of semantic processing assessment in expressive modalities is that of nonverbal capacities like drawing or the execution of meaningful gestures, which are often adopted in treatment (see Sect. 4.6). In PWA after a stroke, drawing tests have been used to assess object representations (Gainotti et al., 1983) and the production of pantomime of object use as limb apraxia assessment (Goldenberg, 2017; van Nispen et al., 2016), but seldom in standardized tests. One recent attempt in that direction is the Nonverbal Semantics Test (NVST; Hogrefe et al., 2022), which comprises Semantic Sorting, Drawing, and Pantomime for the clinical assessment of semantic processing disorders in persons with neurological disorders (cerebrovascular accident [CVA] and neurodegenerative disease).

4.6   Application and Therapeutic Approaches

Because the impairment on word classes is very debilitating in non-fluent or anomic patients, much attention has been devoted in treatments to rehabilitate word retrieval. Several types of intervention have been developed that target the enhancement of the processes underlying the operation, as well as the neural regions where these take place (Raymer & Roitsch, 2023) and have overall been found to be successful in enhancing word naming (Wisenburn & Mahoney, 2009). The treatment approaches usually employ different types of cues, mostly either semantic, phonological, or mixed cues, and vary on the succession of presentation of stimuli and type of feedback provided.

Cues can be either verbal or non-verbal in nature, and they can be of several kinds. For example, categorical cues are words or objects that belong to the same category of words as the target word; similarly, phonemic cues are words that share some phonetic traits with the target word.

In hierarchical treatments, specificity is gradually added to the instructions as the patient tries to recall a word (see Table 4.1, an example from Linebaugh et al., 2005). In the example in Table 4.1, which employs semantic cues, the patient is first guided by concept associations (1–4), then by the semantic and syntactic context (6), and finally aided in the phonetic completion of the word (7–10).

Table 4.1 A cueing hierarchy (adapted from Linebaugh et al., 2005)

1	"What is this called?"
2	Directions to state the function of the item
3	Directions to demonstrate the function
4	Statement of the function by the clinician
5	Statement and demonstration of the function by the clinician
6	Sentence completion
7	Sentence completion + the silently articulated first phoneme of the response
8	Sentence completion + the vocalized first phoneme
9	Sentence completion + the first two phonemes vocalized
10	Say "_____"

Typically, cues are given when a mistake is made in word retrieval.

Despite the known occurrence of impairments in verbs, and in verb inflection specifically, fewer treatments have been proposed to address this impairment (reviewed in Valinejad et al., 2022). In the morphosemantic treatment developed by Faroqi-Shah (2008), patients are aided in morphology production with a process of association between a temporal adverb (such as yesterday) and temporal morphology (in this case, past morphology). After a test of naming, where the patient is asked to name the action taking place in a three-panel picture, he/she is trained to spot sentences with a mismatch between temporal adverb and temporal morphology in auditorily presented sentences, as well as to match the correct temporal morphology to the correct picture, before being asked to complete sentenced with verbs with the correct verb morphology.

Semantically-based treatments, such as Semantic Feature Analysis treatment (SFA; Boyle & Coelho, 1995) and semantic feature verification treatments (Kiran et al., 2009; Kiran & Thompson, 2003), have been proven efficient not only in improving accuracy on trained items, but also in facilitating generalization to untrained items, namely to increase the strength of activation of other words (Evans et al., 2021). In semantically based treatments, participants are guided in the naming of objects through accessing semantically-related concepts. In one treatment, for instance, patients are asked to name a word (picture naming) and are subsequently presented with a card for the target word and cards showing target and non-target semantic features that the patient is asked to select (for example chicken – lays eggs) and asked yes/no questions about the target object. Then the patient is asked to name the object again (Kiran et al., 2009; Kiran & Thompson, 2003).

Aside from treatments of semantic deficits that make use of semantic concepts, other interesting approaches are emerging to the treatment of semantic deficits in aphasia, and particularly naming deficits. One such example is the employment of gesture and combined verbal and gesture treatments. *Gesture treatments*, such as the one described in Rose (2006), make use of non-linguistic communicative devices. Gestures are spontaneous movements of hands and limbs while talking that are argued to have specific meaning in the flow of speech.

4.7   SUMMARY

Semantic aphasia is characterized by selective impairments that may be linked to specific semantic phenomena. In this chapter, we discussed asymmetries in lexical retrieval that are influenced by different properties. Firstly, we discussed how word class has an influence on naming impairments: verb retrieval is often more impaired than noun retrieval in anomic patients. This may be due to a higher processing cost of verbs over nouns. Secondly, we discussed semantic properties of the words, so-called semantic traits. The fact that the effects of these traits may be isolated has been questioned, both for methodological reasons, namely because it is difficult to directly test one property of a word and exclude all others (Capitani et al., 2003), and because several non-linguistic cognitive abilities may be at play (Nickels et al., 2022). However, the asymmetries are reported quite robustly, and we can therefore assume that, within a preexisting impairment in lexical access, some characteristics make the connections harder to establish than others. Incidentally, asymmetries in semantic features are also reported in child language, where some semantic traits are suggested to be learned before others. Without wanting to draw conclusions on the nature of the semantic impairment in aphasia, we might take this as further indication that some traits require higher linguistic abilities than others. In this chapter, we also discussed a semantic characteristic of predicates, which, when featuring a copula construction, may be denoting characteristics of the subject (IP) or of the situation the subject is in (SP). This results, as we have seen, in another asymmetry, where SP show higher omission rates of the copula than IP.

Apart from lexical nouns and verbs, another discourse referent that is highly utilized in any language is deixis, namely the linguistic elements that allow us to refer to highly accessible elements without having to always repeat lexical nouns. Managing deixis is a highly specialized function of human language, and it requires the ability to process the linguistic discourse, the accessibility of all referents, and the choice of words all at the same time. We discussed how this ability may also be impaired in PWA, who will often show difficulties both in using pronouns and in understanding coreference between pronouns and what they refer to.

4.8   Discussion Topics

1. Word naming is severely impaired in anomic patients. Describe what it consists of with examples from studies of people with aphasia and discuss how word naming impairments are treated.
2. Some semantic traits make lexical retrieval harder in PWA. Discuss what these are.
3. What can happen in semantic aphasia with use of deixis? Provide examples from different deictic elements.
4. Temporal morphology on verbs can be selectively omitted. Discuss the distinction between predicates in the verb *to be* and the implications for the study of verbs in PWA.
5. Discuss word retrieval in the case of bilingual aphasia by looking at data on semantic features.
6. Present some examples of semantic-based therapy from a linguistic and an extralinguistic perspective.

References

Arabatzi, M., & Edwards, S. (2002). Tense and syntactic processes in agrammatic speech. *Brain and Language, 80*(3), 314–327.

Bastiaanse, R., Edwards, S., Mass, E., & Rispens, J. (2003). Assessing comprehension and production of verbs and sentences: The Verb and Sentence Test (VAST). *Aphasiology, 17*(1), 49–73.

Becker, M. (2002). The development of the copula in child English: The lightness of be. *Annual Review of Language Acquisition, 2*(1), 37–58.

Becker, M. (2004). Copula omission is a grammatical reflex. *Language Acquisition, 12*(2), 157–167.

Bi, Y., Han, Z., Shu, H., & Caramazza, A. (2007). Nouns, verbs, objects, actions, and the animate/inanimate effect. *Cognitive Neuropsychology, 24*(5), 485–504. https://doi.org/10.1080/02643290701502391

Bialystok, E. (2009). Bilingualism: The good, the bad, and the indifferent. *Bilingualism: Language and Cognition, 12*(1), 3–11.

Boyle, M., & Coelho, C. A. (1995). Application of semantic feature analysis as a treatment for aphasic dysnomia. *American Journal of Speech-Language Pathology, 4*(4), 94–98.

Calabria, M., Grunden, N., Serra, M., García-Sánchez, C., & Costa, A. (2019). Semantic processing in bilingual aphasia: Evidence of language dependency. *Frontiers in Human Neuroscience, 13,* 205.

Capitani, E., Laiacona, M., Mahon, B., & Caramazza, A. (2003). What are the facts of semantic category specific deficits? A critical review of the clinical evidence. *Cognitive Neuropsychology, 20,* 213–261.

Carlson, G. N. (1977). *References to kinds in English.* PhD dissertation. University of Massachusetts.

Chapman, S. B., & Ulatowska, H. K. (1989). Discourse in aphasia: Integration deficits in processing reference. *Brain and Language, 36,* 651–668.

Crepaldi, D. C., Ingignoli, R., Verga, A., Contardi, C. S., & Luzzatti, C. (2011). On nouns, verbs, lexemes, and lemmas: Evidence from the spontaneous speech of seven aphasic patients. *Aphasiology, 25,* 71–92.

Damasio, A. R., & Tranel, D. (1993). Nouns and verbs are retrieved with differently distributed neural systems. *Proceedings of the National Academy of Sciences, 90*(11), 4957–4960.

Evans, W. S., Cavanaugh, E., Gravier, M. L., Autenreith, A. M., Doyle, P. J., Hula, W. D., & Dickey, M. W. (2021). Effects of semantic feature type, diversity, and quality on semantic feature analysis treatment outcomes in aphasia. *American Journal of Speech-Language Pathology, 30,* 344–358.

Faroqi-Shah, Y. (2008). A comparison of two theoretically driven treatments for verb inflection deficits in aphasia. *Neuropsychologia, 46*(13), 3088–3100.

Franklin, S., Howard, D., & Patterson, K. (1995). Abstract word anomia. *Cognitive Neuropsychology, 12*(5), 549–566.

Gainotti, G., Silveri, M. C., Villa, G., & Caltagirone, C. (1983). Drawing objects from memory in aphasia. *Brain, 106*(3), 613–622.

Gleason, J. B., Goodglass, H., Obler, L., Green, E., Hyde, M. R., & Weintraub, S. (1980). Narrative strategies of aphasic and normal-speaking subjects. *Journal of Speech, Language, and Hearing Research, 23*(2), 370–382.

Goldenberg, G. (2017). Facets of pantomime. *Journal of the International Neuropsychological Society, 23*(2), 121–127.

Goodglass, H., Kaplan, E., & Weintraub, S. (2001). BDAE: The Boston diagnostic aphasia examination. Lippincott Williams & Wilkins.

Herbert, R., & Best, W. (2010). The role of noun syntax in spoken word production: Evidence from aphasia. *Cortex, 46*(3), 329–342.

Hogrefe, K., Glindemann, R., Ziegler, W., & Goldenberg, G. (2022). *NVST: nonverbaler Semantiktest.*

Kambanaros, M. (2016). Verb and noun word retrieval in bilingual aphasia: A case study of language- and modality-specific levels of breakdown. *International Journal of Bilingual Education and Bilingualism, 19*(2), 169–184.

Kaplan, E., Goodglass, H., & Weintraub, S. (1983). *The Boston naming test.* Lea & Febiger.

Kay, J., Lesser, R., & Coltheart, M. (1996). Psycholinguistic assessments of language processing in aphasia (PALPA): An introduction. *Aphasiology, 10*(2), 159–180.

Kertesz, A. (2007). *Western aphasia battery-revised.* Grune & Stratton.

Keshree, N. K., Kumar, S., Basu, S., Chakrabarty, M., & Kishore, T. (2013). Adaptation of the Western aphasia battery in Bangla. *Psychology of Language and Communication, 17*(2), 189–201. https://doi.org/10.2478/plc-2013-0012

Kim, H., & Na, D. L. (2004). Normative data on the Korean version of the Western aphasia battery. *Journal of Clinical and Experimental Neuropsychology.* https://doi.org/10.1080/13803390490515397

Kiran, S., Sandberg, C., & Abbott, K. (2009). Treatment for lexical retrieval using abstract and concrete words in persons with aphasia: Effect of complexity. *Aphasiology, 23*(7–8), 835–853.

Kiran, S., & Thompson, C. K. (2003). The role of semantic complexity in treatment of naming deficits. *Journal of Speech, Language, and Hearing Research, 46*(4), 773–787.

Laiacona, M., & Capitani, E. (2001). A case of prevailing deficit of nonliving categories or a case of prevailing sparing of living categories? *Cognitive Neuropsychology, 18*(1), 39–70.

Linebaugh, C. W., Shisler, R. J., & Lehner, L. (2005). CAC classics: Cueing hierarchies and word retrieval: A therapy program. *Aphasiology, 19*(1), 77–92.

Luzzatti, C., Aggujaro, S., & Crepaldi, D. (2006). Noun–verb double dissociation in aphasia: Theoretical and neuroanatomical foundations. *Cortex, 42*, 875–883.

Mahon, B. Z., & Caramazza, A. (2009). Concepts and categories: A cognitive neuropsychological perspective. *Annual Review of Psychology, 60*, 27–51.

Martínez-Ferreiro, S., Ishkhanyan, B., Rosell-Clarí, V., & Boye, K. (2019). Prepositions and pronouns in connected discourse of individuals with aphasia. *Clinical Linguistics & Phonetics, 33*(6), 497–517. https://doi.org/10.1080/02699206.2018.1551935

Miceli, G., Silveri, M. C., Villa, G., & Caramazza, A. (1984). On the basis for the agrammatic's difficulty in producing main verbs. *Cortex, 20*(2), 207–220.

Mirman, D., & Britt, A. E. (2014). What we talk about when we talk about access deficits. *Philosophical Transactions of the Royal Society B: Biological Sciences, 369*, 20120388. https://doi.org/10.1098/rstb.2012.0388

Nickels, L. (2001). *Spoken word production. The handbook of cognitive neuropsychology: What deficits reveal about the human mind* (pp. 291–320). Psychology Press.

Nickels, L., Lampe, L. F., Mason, C., & Hameau, S. (2022). Investigating the influence of semantic factors on word retrieval: Reservations, results and recommendations. *Cognitive Neuropsychology, 39*(3–4), 113–154.

Papagno, C., Capasso, R., & Miceli, G. (2009). Reversed concreteness effect for nouns in a subject with semantic dementia. *Neuropsychologia, 47*(4), 1138–1148.

Parsons, S. D. (1993). *Deixis in aphasic language*. PhD dissertation. University of Texas.

Raymer, A. M., & Roitsch, J. (2023). Effectiveness of constraint-induced language therapy for aphasia: Evidence from systematic reviews and meta-analyses. *American Journal of Speech-Language Pathology, 32*(5S), 2393–2401.

Rose, M. (2006). The utility of arm and hand gestures in the treatment of aphasia. *Advances in Speech-Language Pathology, 8*(2), 92–109.

Shapiro, K., & Caramazza, A. (2003a). The representation of grammatical categories in the brain. *Trends in Cognitive Sciences, 7*(5), 201–206.

Shapiro, K., & Caramazza, A. (2003b). Grammatical processing of nouns and verbs in left frontal cortex? *Neuropsychologia, 41*(9), 1189–1198.

Smith, G., Kershaw, C., Brunetto, V., & Garraffa, M. (2023). 'To be' or not 'to be': An analysis of copula production and omission in people with non-fluent aphasia. *Aphasiology*. https://doi.org/10.1080/02687038.2023.2262687

Tessaro, B., Hameau, S., Salis, C., & Nickels, L. (2022). Semantic impairment in aphasia: A problem of control? *International Journal of Speech-Language Pathology*, 1–12.

Thompson, C. K., Lange, K. L., Schneider, S. L., & Shapiro, L. P. (1997). Agrammatic and non-brain-damaged subjects' verb and verb argument structure production. *Aphasiology, 11*(4–5), 473–490.

Thompson, C. K., Lukic, S., King, M. C., Mesulam, M. M., & Weintraub, S. (2016). Verb and noun deficits in stroke-induced and primary progressive aphasia: The northwestern naming battery. In *The science of aphasia rehabilitation* (pp. 18–41). Routledge.

Ulatowska, H. K., Freedman-Stern, R., Doyel, A. W., Macaluso-Haynes, S., & North, A. J. (1983). Production of narrative discourse in aphasia. *Brain and Language, 19*(2), 317–334.

Valinejad, V., Mehri, A., Khatoonabadi, A., & Shekari, E. (2022). Treatment of verb tense morphology in agrammatic aphasia: A systematic review. *Journal of Neurolinguistics, 62*, 101045.

van Nispen, K., van de Sandt-Koenderman, M., Mol, L., & Krahmer, E. (2016). Pantomime production by people with aphasia: What are influencing factors?. *Journal of Speech, Language, and Hearing Research, 59*(4), 745–758.

Wallace, S. J., Worrall, L., Rose, T., Le Dorze, G., Breitenstein, C., Hilari, K., Babbitt, E., Bose, A., Brady, M., Cherney, L. R., Copland, D., Cruice, M., Enderby, P., Hersh, D., Howe, T., Kelly, H., Kiran, S., Laska, A. C., Marshall, J., Nicholas, M., & Webster, J. (2019). A core outcome set for aphasia treatment research: The ROMA consensus statement. *International Journal of Stroke: Official Journal of the International Stroke Society, 14*(2), 180–185. https://doi.org/10.1177/1747493018806200

Wisenburn, B., & Mahoney, K. (2009). A meta-analysis of word-finding treatments for aphasia. *Aphasiology, 23*(11), 1338–1352.

CHAPTER 5

Disorders of Syntax in Aphasia

Abstract Disorders of syntax in patients with aphasia have been found in both sentence comprehension and production, in relation to how the words are combined into larger units and some specific omissions of elements needed to integrate words into sentences. These include difficulties with sentences that require the correct interpretation of verb morphology (e.g., passive clauses, and other affixes) or sentences with a different order of words that requires more processing for the information to be understood (e.g., non-canonical sentence with a OSV order). In this chapter, we will discuss some relevant outcomes of research in syntax in aphasia, what these entail for a syntactic disorder, sometimes called agrammatism, and some implications for clinical protocols based on sentence level recovery.

Keywords Subject–verb agreement • Argument structure • Relative clauses • Passive clauses • Reversibility • Treatment of underlying form

5.1 Introducing Syntax in Aphasia

Unlike other areas of language, syntactic theory and aphasiology have been in dialogue and informed each other for decades (see Garraffa & Fyndanis 2020 for a recent overview). Nevertheless, the disorder of syntax, sometimes referred to as "agrammatism", is to this day hardly addressed in clinical practice. But what are we talking about when we talk about syntax? When we utter a sentence, we describe a scene that is either imagined or in front of our eyes. At the center of that scene is an event that is taking place. The semantic information of these events is normally coded in the verb. The verb *sing*, for example, contains semantic information around the nature of the action, which in this case is the modulation of vocal cords in a way that produces a musical sound. Oftentimes, this semantic information is contained in a larger portion of language containing the verb, which is referred to as **verb phrase**. An example of a verb phrase is, for example, *singing a number*, where to express the semantics of the action to the fullest, the verb comes with a grammatical object (*number*). The examples seen here are verbs or verb phrases in isolation. As we can see from the example *sing* and *singing a number*, verb and verb phrases in isolation cannot describe world events directly, and so they do not constitute a sentence by themselves. They still need to express the "doer," who is doing the action of singing. This is called the grammatical subject, and it is a necessary component for a unit to be defined as a sentence.

Within sentences, verb phrases with subjects convey the role(s) of the actors in the event, see examples in (1) from English.

(1) a. **The girl** smiled.
    b. **The birds** were singing.
    c. **I** am walking along the river.
    d. **He** was walking his dog.

Syntax is the area of language governing the relations between elements of a sentence. As we will see in the following sections, there are several of these relations that can be impaired in aphasia. These are related to the verb and its arguments (Sect. 5.2), the verb and its subject (Sect. 5.3), and the whole structure of the sentence (Sect. 5.4).

5.2   Argument Structure

Any verb that functions as the kernel of a sentence needs to have a structure. The argument structure of a verb indicates its *configuration*, namely which elements (*arguments*) need to be realized for the meaning and the syntax of the predicate to be satisfied. The possible arguments are subjects and any direct or indirect object.

Intransitive verbs such as *fall* only need one argument, namely the subject (*She fell*), while transitive verbs require a subject and one or more objects (*She read the book, Mary bought Mark some flowers*). Argument structure has been proposed to have a role for aphasic speakers in verb retrieval, which we discussed in opposition to noun retrieval in Chap. 4. A first result in this sense is that people with aphasia are facilitated in the production of complete syntactic sentences when the verb of the sentence has fewer arguments. The pattern proposed for people with aphasia is that they retrieve more accurately the argument structure of intransitive verbs (verbs with one obligatory argument), followed by ditransitive verbs (verbs with two obligatory arguments), followed by tritransitive verbs (verbs with three obligatory arguments) (Argument Structure Complexity Hypothesis, Thompson, 2003). Thompson et al. (1997) investigated the effects of different argument structures on verb production in ten agrammatic and ten control participants. The participants were presented with three tasks: picture naming, story completion, and sentence production. The authors found that one-argument verbs were easier to produce than two-argument ones, and that these, in turn, were easier than three-argument verbs across tasks. Not all the differences, however, were significant. Kim and Thompson (2000) replicated this result in another group of patients, and they found that the hierarchy is not only visible when people with aphasia are asked to produce full sentences, but even in single-word retrieval, namely when they are asked to retrieve the verb alone without its arguments. The perceived difficulty with these multi-argumental verbs is therefore not only linked to the production of more constituents. The results found for English have been replicated cross-linguistically, for instance in German (De Bleser & Kauschke, 2003) and Hungarian (Kiss, 2001).

Perhaps even more interestingly, another distinction has been detected within intransitive verbs, supposedly the easiest verbs in the hierarchy. Among intransitive verbs, there are two syntactic classes: unergatives, such as *sleep* (2a), and unaccusatives, such as *melt* (2b).

(2) a. The baby is sleeping.
    b. Ice melts.

In the case of unergative verbs like (2a), the subject of the verb is also the thematic agent, and the structure of the verb phrase is therefore very simple: [V]. The sentence is ready: NP [V]. In the case of unaccusatives, the subject of the verb is not its agent but its *theme*. In (2b) above, melt is an action that ice undergoes, not the action that ice undertakes. Therefore, the structure of the verb phrase is: [V NP], where V is the verb, and NP is its internal argument. In unaccusative verbs, the internal argument becomes the subject of the verb. For this reason, it must move from its originating position to the subject position, like so:

NP [V <NP>].

In a seminal paper investigating the role of the underlying syntactic structure in the production of one-argument verbs, Thompson (2003) found that unergative verbs are produced more easily than unaccusative verbs by speakers with aphasia.

5.3   AGREEMENT

The close link between the verb in a sentence and its subject is visible in the expression of an **agreement** between the subject and the verb. We can see instances of *number* agreement in examples (1b–d) above. In these examples, the verb is composite containing an auxiliary *be*, which agrees in number with the subject: in (1b) it is plural, like *birds were*, in (1c–d) it is singular, like subject pronouns *I am* and *he was*.

Efficient grammatical processing depends on the integration of the morphological information of subject and verb. We have seen in Chap. 3 that there is converging evidence suggesting that the production of number Subject–Verb agreement is generally preserved in patients with aphasia (Friedmann & Grodzinsky, 1997; Clahsen & Ali, 2009). The same is true for comprehension, with some differences for conditions relying more heavily on cognitive load (Kok et al., 2007). To check whether this holds true in situations where finer grained syntactic abilities are in place, grammatical agreement has been investigated in the condition of **attraction**. Attraction occurs when there is a linguistic element, for example a prepositional phrase, intervening between the verb and the subject. When the morphological features of the element are morphologically different from that of the subject (feature *mismatch* condition), it is said that these can *attract* agreement (Bock & Miller, 1991). An example of attraction is given in (3). Attraction is considerably more likely to occur when an intervener is grammatically plural than when it is singular (an effect of plural *markedness*).

(3) *The coat with the red buttons *are* on the coat hanger.

In (3) the plural of *red buttons* is still active and mapped on the verb that should be singular as the subject is *the coat*.

Interestingly, studies have shown that PWA are generally more prone to attraction errors than healthy participants are. Vigliocco and colleagues (Vigliocco & Zilli, 1999; Vigliocco et al., 1994) found attraction effects of greater magnitude in two Italian-speaking PWA over controls. More recently, a similar effect was found in three out of four PWA speakers of English (Slevc & Martin, 2016). The effects of sensitivity to both syntactic and semantic factors in agreement errors, as well as the role of cognitive load on working memory, are debated.

Importantly, some effects of attraction have also been found in comprehension. In a case study, a 42-year-old female non-fluent PWA speaker of Italian was tested on agreement attraction in different subject–verb agreements (Garraffa, 2009). The participant showed very few errors of agreement in spontaneous speech as well as in a completion task with no interveners, findings consistent with the results reviewed so far. A series of grammaticality judgement task-presenting sentences with and without errors of attraction were administered to the patient. The sentences with a potential source of attraction (i.e., an intervener) were either following a Subject–Verb order, or a Verb–Subject order, both of which are plausible in Italian, as shown in (8a, 8b) below:

(8) a. L'autista dei ministri guida/*guidano con prudenza. (SV)
    b. Guida/*guidano con prudenza l'autista dei ministri. (VS)
    The driver of the ministers drives/*drive with caution.

The participant showed effects of attraction on grammatical sentences, which she deemed ungrammatical more frequently than healthy controls. Consistently, she frequently accepts ungrammatical sentences, displaying around or below chance performance in accuracy in the ungrammatical conditions. As a side note, the highest error rate was in the ungrammatical inverted condition (*VS), suggesting that the position of the subject with respect to the verb is crucial in agreement. Specifically, agreement relations that involve the establishment of a connection between the preverbal position and the post-verbal subject involve a more complex syntactic operation, therefore suggesting that PWA may have a harder time accessing harder computations. See Garraffa (2009) for a detailed discussion on attraction and position of the subject.

5.4   COMPLEX SENTENCES: PASSIVES AND RELATIVE CLAUSES

Consider the following sentences:

(5) The boy that the girl is kicking is tall
(6) The ball that the girl is kicking is red

In their pioneering study, which is widely cited as initiating research on sentence comprehension deficits in aphasia, Caramazza and Zurif (1976) find that patients with Broca's aphasia perform well in a sentence comprehension task in sentences like (6), but at chance in sentences like (5). In sentence–picture comprehension tasks, participants are presented with two (sometimes up to four) images together with an orally or written presented sentence. Participants are asked to judge which of the pictures describes the sentence. In the case of (5), the target picture of a girl kicking a (tall) boy is presented with a competitor picture in which a (tall) boy is kicking a girl. What is the difference between (5) and (6)? The sentence in (5) is *semantically reversible*; the sentence in (6) is not. What is meant by reversible is that the participants involved in the action do not give us an indication of *who is doing what to whom*: the action of kicking can be performed by both the girl and the (tall) boy. Conversely, in the world as we know it, only a girl can kick a ball and not vice versa.

This becomes of crucial importance in the interpretation of *passive sentences*. In the reversible active sentence in (7), the Subject of the verb is the agent performing the action of kissing. Conversely, in the reversible passive sentence in (8), the Subject of the sentence is *not* the one performing the action of kissing.

(7) The little girl is kissing the cook.
(8) The little girl is being kissed by the cook.

Figure 5.1 shows a typical example of picture selection (or sentence–picture matching) task for active and passive sentences. If participants hear sentence (7), they are expected to select Fig. 5.1b. If they hear sentence (8), they should select Fig. 5.1a. To correctly interpret reversible sentences, where no semantic cue is available to understand to establish who is doing what to whom, one must be able to access the syntactic structure of the sentence.

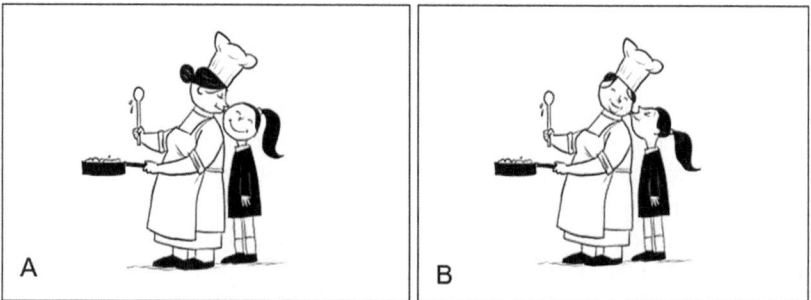

Fig. 5.1 A picture adopted in the studies of reversible sentences

The comprehension of (reversible) passives has been robustly shown to be impaired in people with aphasia with difficulties in syntax (e.g., Berndt et al., 1997; Friederici & Graetz, 1987; Goodglass, 1993; Goodglass et al., 1993; Grodzinsky, 2000). This selective difficulty is the result of difficulties in the processing of thematic roles and/or of the specific syntactic structure of passive sentences (see Druks, 2016 for considerations on existing accounts and Beber et al., 2024 for a recent systematic review of thematic impairments in aphasia).

Similar results have been attested in production as well. In tasks eliciting the production of passives, participants are typically shown a picture, like Fig. 5.1b, and are asked to formulate a sentence describing the picture. Cues are given on how to start the sentence, as exemplified in the examples below (9a and 9b):

(9a) The little girl ... (prompt for active sentence)
(9b) The cook ... (prompt for passive sentence)

In production, agrammatic speakers have been shown to make errors when producing passives which include the omission of the grammatical morphemes related to passives (e.g., in English the auxiliary and 'by' (Caplan & Hanna, 1998)) and the inversion of the roles of the agent and patient (Bastiaanse & Edwards, 2004; Caramazza & Berndt, 1985; Benedet et al., 1998). It is important to mention that the difficulty with passives has been found cross-linguistically, but it is not generalizable to all passives. For example, the active/passive asymmetry has not been detected in Indonesian and Malay, two languages that heavily rely on affixation to determine the roles of the participants in the event. Aziz et al. (2020, 2024) confronted the comprehension of reversible active and passive sentences with varying number or arguments in a sentence–picture matching task. The authors found participants to perform worse than controls overall, but to show no asymmetry across sentence type (active/passive). Interestingly, an asymmetry was only visible in error types, with thematic role reversal errors predominantly occurring in passive sentences. The authors conclude that the difficulty likely lies at the level of affix processing (see Chap. 3), thereby generating from under specification of the grammatical features.

In Sect. 5.3, we saw that the intervention of linguistic material between a verb and its subject may pose difficulties to PWA, particularly when this linguistic material mismatches in features with the Subject. Another structure where the intervention of linguistic material creates a source of difficulty is the relative clause. Relative clauses are understood to be the result of movement of the noun in brackets < >, which has an originating position and role.

(10a) Mary talked to the girl. The girl is kissing her mother.
Mary talked to the girl that <the girl> is kissing her mother.
(10b) Mary talked to the mother. The girl is kissing the mother.
Mary talked to the mother that the girl is kissing <the mother>.

(10a) is a subject relative clause because the element in brackets is in subject position in the relative clause between square brackets. (10b) is an object relative clause. It is a known phenomenon in psycholinguistics that the processing of object relative clauses, as in (10b), can be more demanding than the processing of subject relative clauses, as attested in acquisition, developmental language disorders, and aphasia. In fact, agrammatic speakers have been shown to present a selective vulnerability in the comprehension and production of object relative clauses over subject relative clauses (e.g., Berndt & Caramazza, 1980; Caramazza & Zurif, 1976; Schwartz et al., 1980; Garraffa & Grillo, 2008). Garraffa and Grillo (2008), working on the theoretical framework of canonicity developed in Grillo (2003, 2005, and later 2009), propose this to be the result of intervention and more visible if the two nouns share features. The term intervention refers to the difficulty in establishing a syntactic relation (called a *dependency* in syntax) when the two terms of the relation are separated by an intervening element, an element that can potentially enter in the same relation with the two elements. In the case of object relative clauses, the subject of the relative clause (in (10b) *the girl*) intervenes in the relation between the object of the matrix clause (*the mother*) and the information about its position in the relative clause (*<the mother>*).

Syntactic priming in aphasia: Syntactic or structural priming is a phenomenon that can be described as a facilitation of using a certain sentence if still active in a conversation (see Garraffa & Smith (2022) for an overview on syntactic priming as a tool to investigate atypical language). Priming effects have been reported in many languages and in different populations, to elicit the production of sentences which may be difficult to encounter in certain speakers such as in PWA. Priming effects are those which determine that exposure to a specific word or structure will influence the way we process language and might determine our linguistic behavior in the following moments. For example, if we hear someone use the structure "Give John the ball" instead of "Give the ball to John," we are more likely to use the structure that was used before ourselves even if for example more complex and not frequent in the input.

This paradigm is currently being used more and more to explore the language of atypical speakers, thanks to its power to identify whether the structures are accessible in any way. A few studies have applied the syntactic priming paradigm to investigate whether priming effects can be elicited in PWA, and whether they are comparable with the one reported for healthy subjects. Priming effects were not only found in both PWA and healthy controls, even when four intervening sentences were placed between prime and target sentence, but PWA exhibit an even stronger priming effect compared to healthy subjects (Cho-Reyes et al., 2016). Priming effects in this population appear regardless of whether or not there is a lexical boost, namely when the reuse of the structure is boosted by using some of the same words, as was shown in a study where sentences with and without lexical overlap between the primed sentence and the target sentence were included (Lee et al., 2019). This result indicates that the priming effect is, in fact, activating abstract representations of the primed structures, as is also supported by the fact that priming effects in PWA can be long-term in nature.

The same framework has been proposed for the similar pattern found in children (Adani, 2011).

Further asymmetries within Object Relative Clauses (ORCs) have been discovered, which are again dependent on the intervention of linguistic material. Much like with subject–verb agreement, in this case what is crucial is the **features** of the intervening material. The principle of featural Relativized Minimality (Friedmann et al., 2009) predicts that an impairment of grammar will be visible when there is a match in features between two elements of the relative clause. The prediction has been borne out in several studies with PWA, for instance in Greek (Terzi & Nanousi, 2018) and Italian (Martini et al., 2020). Terzi & Nanousi found that six non-fluent Greek-speaking PWA performed worse on ORCs than SRCs, and that within ORCs, sentences where the subject of the matrix sentence and that of the RC have the same gender, as in (11), are harder than those where the two nouns have different genders, as in (12).

(11) Dhikse mu **ti vasilisa** pu akoluthi **i kiria** (ORC same gender)

Show me the queen (fem., accusative) that follows the lady (fem., nominative)
"Show me the queen that the lady follows"

(12) Dhikse mu **ti jaja** pu fotoghrafizi **o ghabros** (ORC different gender)

Show me the grandmother (fem., acc.) that photographs the groom (masc., nom.)
"Show me the grandmother that the groom photographs"

5.5   Assessments of Syntax for Aphasia

We have seen in previous sections that a disorder in syntax, namely one at the level of sentence construction or processing, can vary depending on the modality (comprehension and production) and, within the same set of sentences, on the specific properties of a subset of sentences (for example, reversible passives, sentences with interveners with a mismatch in features between the subject and the verb, sentences with interveners with a match in features between the object of the matrix and its originating position in the relative clause, and so on). Therefore, it is intuitive to see that assessing a disorder of syntax is not straightforward. Several standardized measures exist for the English language, which capitalize on different aspects of sentence production and/or comprehension.

Both the *Western Aphasia Battery* (WAB; Kertesz, 1982) and the *Boston Diagnostic Aphasia Examination* (BDAE; Goodglass et al., 2001) examine sentence production in narrative speech. Sentences tested for comprehension include simple yes/no questions and imperative sentences, and there is no specific distinction between types of sentences, and sentence production and the comprehension of non-canonical sentences is not included.

The *Comprehensive Aphasia Test* (CAT; Swinburn et al., 2004) and the *Northwestern Assessment of Verbs and Sentences* (NAVS; Thompson, 2011), on the other hand, test a series of non-canonical sentences, from passives to object relatives. The NAVS, in particular, assesses passives and object relatives in both production and comprehension tasks.

An honorable mention goes to the *Bilingual Aphasia Test* (BAT; Paradis & Libben, 2014), which was designed to assess each of the languages of a bilingual or multilingual individual with aphasia in an equivalent way, and has several adaptations as well as language pairs.

5.6   APPLICATIONS IN APHASIA
AND THERAPEUTIC APPROACHES

In this section, we will be presenting two therapeutic interventions that target syntax for aphasia: one that targets verbs and verb argument structure (Loverso et al., 1992; Edmonds, 2016; Thompson et al. 2013), and one that targets complex structures (Thompson & Shapiro, 2005).

Studies for verb retrieval have focused on the remediation of both semantic (e.g., Raymer & Ellsworth, 2002) and phonological impairments (e.g., Fink et al., 1993). These therapies have generally resulted in improved production of the treated verbs but no improvement in the production of untrained verbs. There have been a more limited number of therapy studies explicitly targeting argument structure. For example, after the naming of the verb, Fink et al. (1993), in their "direct verb training," asked the client to generate the agent and theme before producing a sentence to describe. Perhaps the most successful treatment of verbs is the Verb Argument Structure Treatment (Thompson et al., 2013). This treatment consists of sessions of production of three-argument verbs in sentence contexts until patients reach 80% accuracy, followed by probe tasks, testing all trained verbs as well as a subset of untrained (two- and one-argument) verbs. During training sessions, line drawings for three-argument verbs are presented together with a sentence production template consisting of place-holders for all verb arguments and the target verb.

The Treatment of Underlying Forms (TUF) (Thompson & Shapiro, 2005) is a linguistically based intervention approach to agrammatic aphasia. The TUF focuses on syntactically complex structures such as sentences with non-canonical ORCs (e.g., "The man saw the artist who the thief chased") rather than on simple (canonical) sentences (e.g., "The man saw the artist"). Several studies by Thompson and colleagues (e.g., Ballard & Thompson, 1999; Thompson et al., 1993, 1998) report evidence that training structurally complex sentences results in greater generalization to untrained (but structurally/linguistically related) sentences as compared with training fewer complex sentences. To explain these findings, Thompson (2003) proposed the Complexity Account of Treatment Efficacy, which posits that training structurally complex sentences results in generalization to fewer complex sentences only "when untreated structures encompass processes relevant to (i.e., are in a subset relation to) treated ones" (Thompson, 2003, p. 602). For example, training complex sentences such as *The man saw the artist who the thief chased* (i.e., a two-proposition sentence with an object-extracted relative clause) results in generalization to untreated structurally related fewer complex sentences such as *It was the artist who the thief chased* (object cleft sentence) and *Who did the thief chase?* (Object wh-question). What the three sentences above have in common is that they involve wh-movement and object extraction. However, they differ in complexity because they also involve other operations. Without going into specific details, sentences with object-extracted relative clauses are more complex than object cleft sentences. Given the difference above, and since the syntactic process taking place in matrix object questions is identical to the syntactic process occurring in the relative clauses of the two more complex sentences described above, the syntactic structure of matrix object questions is a subset of the syntactic structure of sentences with object-extracted relative clauses and object cleft sentences (again, for more details see Thompson & Shapiro, 2005; also see Thompson 2019, for review).

TUF treatments are founded in a metalinguistic approach, pushing agrammatic aphasics to find and utilize the schemes underlying sentence production and comprehension that come naturally to the healthy speaker. In the first phase, PWA undergoing TUF receive a training in the production and comprehension of the constituents of the non-canonical sentences (Thompson & Shapiro, 2005). This is done by observing canonical sentences, drawing the patient's attention towards aspects of the constituents such as the observation of the thematic role information around verbs (Thompson, 2003). Then, explicit instructions on the syntactic operations (movement) that allow for the creation of non-canonical sentences starting from canonical ones are given by means of cards containing the written constituents, that are moved around in front of the patient so as to mimic the operation. The patient is then trained in the comprehension and production of non-canonical sentences. Increase in performance using TUF treatments, as proven by the increase in accuracy not only on the trained sentences, but also on untrained sentences, is robust in the literature, as is nicely demonstrated in a recent meta-analysis by Swiderski et al. (2021).

5.7   Summary

In this chapter we have discussed impairments in grammar in PWA. We have seen that PWA have difficulties compared to controls in both the production and the comprehension of specific sentence types. Importantly, the fact that these asymmetries between types of sentences are also present in comprehension confirms that impairments in grammar are not only limited to difficulties in producing sentences tout court, but are also rooted in the syntactic nature of specific constructions. This is also shown by further asymmetries such as the one we discussed for ORCs with a number match, where the specific properties of the elements involved in the derivation, in this case the features of the elements, have different predictions on the complexity of the structures. Overall, we can say that agrammatism is a phenomenon that has attracted a lot of attention in linguistic theory given its strict relationship with grammatic structures; however, it is important that it is not overlooked in clinical settings either. As it is limited to the more complex structures of language, it is, unlike types of aphasia that occur in frequent elements such as anomia, harder to recognize, as patients will often be able to recover by using simpler language. Consequently, theory-informed assessments of language that cover all possible pockets of impairment must be adopted.

5.8   Discussion Topics

1. Explain the role of argument structure in determining the outcomes of lexical retrieval in PWA.
2. What is reversibility? Explain why reversible passives are harder than reversible actives in English.
3. Construct some examples of agreement between subject and verb with intervening material.
4. Construct some ORCs in English that have matched and mismatched features and discuss the reason why the matched features ones are more complex.
5. Develop a short list of sentences that you think are "easy," and a short list of sentences that you think are "hard," and justify your decisions.

References

Adani, F. (2011). Rethinking the acquisition of relative clauses in Italian: Towards a grammatically based account. *Journal of Child Language, 38*(1), 141–165.

Aziz, A., Smith, G., & Garraffa, M. (2024). Sentence comprehension in Malay-speaking adults with aphasia: The role of affix integration. *Aphasiology.* Special issue on "Across countries, cultures and languages: Assessing aphasia in diverse clinical populations." https://doi.org/10.1080/02687038.2024.2406577.

Aziz, M. A. A., Hassan, M., Razak, R. A., & Garraffa, M. (2020). Syntactic abilities in Malay adult speakers with aphasia: A study on passive sentences and argument structures. *Aphasiology, 34*(7), 886–904.

Ballard, K. J., & Thompson, C. K. (1999). Treatment and generalization of complex sentence production in agrammatism. *Journal of Speech, Language, and Hearing Research, 42*(3), 690–707.

Bastiaanse, R., & Edwards, S. (2004). Word order and finiteness in Dutch and English Broca's and Wernicke's aphasia. *Brain and Language, 89,* 91–107.

Beber, S., Bontempi, G., Miceli, G., & Tettamanti, M. (2024). The Neurofunctional correlates of Morphosyntactic and thematic impairments in aphasia: A systematic review and meta-analysis. *Neuropsychology Review,* 1–34.

Benedet, M. J., Christiansen, J. A., & Goodglass, H. (1998). A cross-linguistic study of grammatical morphology in Spanish- and English-speaking agrammatic patients. *Cortex, 34,* 309–336.

Berndt, R. S., & Caramazza, A. (1980). A redefinition of the syndrome of Broca's aphasia: Implications for a neuropsychological model of language. *Applied Psycholinguistics, 1*(3), 225–278.

Berndt, R. S., Mitchum, C. C., & Wayland, S. (1997). Patterns of sentence comprehension in aphasia: A consideration of three hypotheses. *Brain and Language, 60*(2), 197–221.

Bock, K., & Miller, C. A. (1991). Broken agreement. *Cognitive Psychology, 23*(1), 45–93.

Caplan, D., & Hanna, J. (1998). Sentence production by aphasic patients in a constrained task. *Brain and Language, 63*, 184–218.

Caramazza, A., & Berndt, R. S. (1985). A multicomponent deficit view of agrammatic Broca's aphasia. In M. L. Kean (Ed.), *Agrammatism*. Academic Press.

Caramazza, A., & Zurif, E. B. (1976). Dissociation of algorithmic and heuristic processes in language comprehension: Evidence from aphasia. *Brain and Language, 3*(4), 572–582.

Cho-Reyes, S., Mack, J. E., & Thompson, C. K. (2016). Grammatical encoding and learning in agrammatic aphasia: Evidence from structural priming. *Journal of Memory and Language, 91*, 202–218.

Clahsen, H., & Ali, M. (2009). Formal features in aphasia: Tense, agreement, and mood in English agrammatism. *Journal of Neurolinguistics, 22*(5), 436–450.

De Bleser, R., & Kauschke, C. (2003). Acquisition and loss of nouns and verbs: Parallel or divergent patterns?. *Journal of Neurolinguistics, 16*(2–3), 213–229.

Druks, J. (2016). *Contemporary and emergent theories of Agrammatism: A neurolinguistic approach*. Routledge.

Edmonds, L. A. (2016). A review of Verb Network Strengthening Treatment: Theory, methods, results, and clinical implications. *Topics in Language Disorders, 36*(2), 123–135.

Fink, R. B., Martin, N., Schwartz, M. F., Saffron, E. M., & Myers, J. L. (1993). Facilitation of verb retrieval skills in aphasia: A comparison of two approaches. *Clinical Aphasiology, 21*, 263–272.

Friederici, A. D., & Graetz, P. A. (1987). Processing passive sentences in aphasia: Deficits and strategies. *Brain and Language, 30*(1), 93–105. https://doi.org/10.1016/0093-934X(87)90030-7

Friedmann, N., Belletti, A., & Rizzi, L. (2009). Relativized relatives: Types of intervention in the acquisition of A-bar dependencies. *Lingua, 119*, 67–88. https://doi.org/10.1016/j.lingua.2008.09.002

Friedmann, N. A., & Grodzinsky, Y. (1997). Tense and agreement in agrammatic production: Pruning the syntactic tree. *Brain and Language, 56*(3), 397–425.

Garraffa, M. (2009). Minimal structures in aphasia: A study on agreement and movement in a non-fluent aphasic speaker. *Lingua, 119*(10), 1444–1457.

Garraffa, M., & Fyndanis, V. (2020). Linguistic theory and aphasia: An overview. *Aphasiology, 34*(8), 905–926.

Garraffa, M., & Grillo, N. (2008). Canonicity effects as grammatical phenomena. *Journal of Neurolinguistics, 21*(2), 177–197.

Garraffa, M., & Smith, G. (2022). Syntactic priming as a window to investigate grammatical learning in non-typical populations. Syntactic priming in language acquisition: *Representations, mechanisms and applications*, 183–202.

Goodglass, H. (1993). *Understanding aphasia*. Academic Press.

Goodglass, H., Christiansen, J. A., & Gallagher, R. (1993). Comparison of morphology and syntax in free narrative and structured tests: Fluent vs. nonfluent aphasics. *Cortex, 29*(3), 377–407. https://doi.org/10.1016/S0010-9452(13)80250-X

Goodglass, H., Kaplan, E., & Barresi, B. (2001). *The assessment of aphasia and related disorders* (3rd ed.). Lippincott, Williams, & Wilkins.

Grillo, N. (2003). *Comprensione agrammatica tra processing e rappresentazione: effetti di minimalità*. Master's Thesis. Università di Siena.

Grillo, N. (2005). Minimality effects in agrammatic comprehension. In S. Blaho, E. Schoorlemmer, L. Vicente (Eds.), *Proceedings of ConSOLE XIII* (pp. 106–120). http://www.sole.leidenuniv.nl/

Grillo, N. (2009). Generalized Minimality: Feature impoverishment and comprehension deficits in agrammatism. *Lingua, 119*, 1426–1443.

Grodzinsky, Y. (2000). The neurology of syntax: Language use without Broca's area. *Behavioral and Brain Sciences, 23*(1), 1–71.

Kertesz, A. (1982). *Western aphasia battery*. Grune & Stratton.

Kim, M., & Thompson, C. K. (2000). Patterns of comprehension and production of nouns and verbs in agrammatism: Implications for lexical organization. *Brain and language, 74*(1), 1–25.

Kiss, K. (2001). Lexical retrieval of complex predicates in an agrammatic aphasic subject's sentence production. *Acta Linguistica Hungarica, 48*(1), 183–216.

Kok, P., van Doorn, A., & Kolk, H. (2007). Inflection and computational load in agrammatic speech. *Brain and Language, 102*(3), 273–283.

Lee, J., Hosokawa, E., Meehan, S., Martin, N., & Branigan, H. (2019). Priming sentence comprehension in aphasia: Effects of lexically independent and specific structural priming. *Aphasiology, 33*(7), 780–802.

Loverso, F. L., Prescott, T. E., & Selinger, M. (1992). Microcomputer treatment applications in aphasiology. *Aphasiology, 6*, 155–163. https://doi.org/10.1080/02687039208248587

Martini, K., Belletti, A., Centorrino, S., & Garraffa, M. (2020). Syntactic complexity in the presence of an intervener: The case of an Italian speaker with anomia. *Aphasiology, 34*(8), 1016–1042. https://doi.org/10.1080/0268703 8.2019.1686744

Paradis, M., & Libben, G. (2014). *The assessment of bilingual aphasia*. Psychology Press.

Raymer, A. M., & Ellsworth, T. A. (2002). Response to contrasting verb retrieval treatments: A case study. *Aphasiology, 16*(10–11), 1031–1045.

Schwartz, M. F., Saffran, E. M., & Marin, O. S. M. (1980). The word order problem in agrammatism: I. Comprehension. *Brain and Language, 10*, 249–262.

Slevc, L. R., & Martin, R. C. (2016). Syntactic agreement attraction reflects working memory processes. *Journal of Cognitive Psychology, 28*(7), 773–790.

Swiderski, A. M., Quique, Y. M., Dickey, M. W., & Hula, W. D. (2021). Treatment of underlying forms: A Bayesian meta-analysis of the effects of treatment and person-related variables on treatment response. *Journal of Speech, Language, and Hearing Research, 64*, 4308–4328.

Swinburn, K., Porter, G., & Howard, D. (2004). *The comprehensive aphasia test.* Psychology Press.

Terzi, A., & Nanousi, V. (2018). Intervention effects in the relative clauses of agrammatics: The role of gender and case. *Glossa: A Journal of General Linguistics, 3*((1)17), 1–23.

Thompson, C. K. (2003). Unaccusative verb production in agrammatic aphasia: The argument structure complexity hypothesis. *Journal of neurolinguistics, 16*(2–3), 151–167.

Thompson, C. K. (2011). *Northwestern assessment of verbs and sentences.* Evanston, IL.

Thompson, C. K. (2019). Neurocognitive recovery of sentence processing in aphasia. *Journal of Speech, Language, and Hearing Research, 62*(11), 3947–3972.

Thompson, C. K., Ballard, K. J., & Shapiro, L. P. (1998). The role of syntactic complexity in training wh-movement structures in agrammatic aphasia: Optimal order for promoting generalization. *Journal of the International Neuropsychological Society, 4*(6), 661–674. https://doi.org/10.1017/S1355617798466141APHASIOLOGY21

Thompson, C. K., Shapiro, L., Kiran, S., & Sobecks, J. (2003). The role of syntactic complexity in treatment of sentence deficits in agrammatic aphasia: The complexity account of treatment efficacy (CATE). *Journal of Speech, Language, and Hearing Research, 46*(3), 591–607. https://doi.org/10.1044/1092-4388(2003/047)

Thompson, C. K., & Shapiro, L. P. (2005). Treating agrammatic aphasia within a linguistic framework: Treatment of underlying forms. *Aphasiology, 19*(10–11), 1021–1036. https://doi.org/10.1080/02687030544000227

Thompson, C. K., Shapiro, L. P., & Roberts, M. (1993). Treatment of sentence production deficits in aphasia: A linguistic-specific approach to wh-interrogative training and generalization. *Aphasiology, 7*(1), 111–133. https://doi.org/10.1080/02687039308249501

Thompson, C. K., Lange, K. L., Schneider, S. L., & Shapiro, L. P. (1997). Agrammatic and non-brain-damaged subjects' verb and verb argument structure production. *Aphasiology, 11*(4–5), 473–490.

Thompson, C. K., Riley, E. A., den Ouden, D. B., Meltzer-Asscher, A., & Lukic, S. (2013). Training verb argument structure production in agrammatic aphasia: Behavioral and neural recovery patterns. *cortex, 49*(9), 2358–2376.

Vigliocco, G., Butterworth, B., Semenza, C., & Fossella, S. (1994). How two aphasic speakers construct subject—Verb agreement. *Journal of Neurolinguistics, 8*(1), 19–25.

Vigliocco, G., & Zilli, T. (1999). Syntactic accuracy in sentence production: The case of gender disagreement in Italian language-impaired and unimpaired speakers. *Journal of Psycholinguistic Research, 28*, 623–648.

CHAPTER 6

Disorders of Pragmatics and Discourse in Aphasia

Abstract The study of discourse comprehension and pragmatic communication abilities in aphasia plays a crucial role in understanding how to support conversations and communication skills in people with aphasia. In this chapter, evidence-based studies on theoretical models of discourse in both oral and written communication will be reviewed, together with the main factors affecting discourse comprehension in aphasia, such as the nature of the implicatures (non-literal meaning) necessary for understanding a short paragraph and the distinction of the type of information involved (implied information or stated information), the study on coherent speech in people with aphasia and investigations on Theory of Mind in adults with acquired disorders.

Future directions in the assessment and treatment of discourse comprehension will be presented, along with some necessary steps in applying theoretical models to support discourse comprehension in people with aphasia.

Keywords Coherence • Implicatures • Reading comprehension • Implicit information • Main ideas • Discourse comprehension • Theory of mind

© The Author(s), under exclusive license to Springer Nature
Switzerland AG 2024
M. Garraffa, G. Smith, *Linguistic Theory for Aphasia*,
https://doi.org/10.1007/978-3-031-77134-7_6

73

6.1   Introducing Pragmatics in Aphasia

The study of richer linguistics elements such as stories, conversations, and long texts in patients with aphasia is intrinsically linked to the investigation of reasoning abilities and to a more fundamental question about which forms of reasoning are related to the medium of a fully functioning language competence. For example, some degrees of grammatical ability are necessary to reason out a problem, a mental operation as one involving **Theory of Mind** (ToM) in tasks aiming at determining the logic connection between the mental states of others, for example their desires or beliefs (Siegal et al., 2001). One interesting avenue for investigation into the relationship between specific language abilities such as grammar and reasoning concerns the study of people who have severe forms of aphasia, for example with an agrammatic profile. It is widely acknowledged that typical cognition is retained in many cases of aphasia (Kertesz, 1988). If the claim is that language propositions supported by grammatical knowledge are necessary for causal reasoning, a natural test is to consider aphasic patients who have a difficulty with language at sentence level in any modality of language use. Similarly, questions of disruption of cognition in aphasia have been addressed through administering tests from non-verbal intelligence scales with no clear rationale as to why language might be implicated in, for example, visuo-spatial problem solving. It is only now that claims of specific forms of language mediation (e.g., language propositions) in specific types of reasoning (e.g., ToM) have been tested. Recent studies have adopted this more focused approach to the relationship of grammar and cognition in aphasia. Some studies have revealed that patients with severe agrammatic aphasia, who have minimal access to propositional language, can understand simple causal reasoning (see Varley & Siegal, 2000 for a single case study of severe aphasia).

By contrast, nonaphasic patients with lesions to the right (non-language-dominant) hemisphere display impaired ToM reasoning, as well as difficulties in understanding sarcasm, jokes, and the conversational implications of questions (Happé et al., 1999). This double dissociation between grammar and cognition supports the idea that grammatical language is neither a necessary nor a sufficient condition for causal reasoning and ToM understanding. It is possible that people with aphasia may have had normal competency in language prior to brain injury; grammar might then be unnecessary for ongoing reasoning as instead it has served to configure reasoning in children who are acquiring simultaneously both language and reasoning skills. However, evidence from children with developmental language disorders (DLD) indicates that these kids succeed as readily as typical children do on ToM tasks and/or other pragmatic tasks, such as those involving **Grice's maxims** (Osman et al., 2011; Rossi, Rossi et al., 2013 for a study in Italian), thus confirming that grammatical competence is not always required for higher-order reasoning. According to this approach, testing discourse-level comprehension in both oral and written materials is essential for any speaker with aphasia without many limitations to the degree of severity of the acquired disorder.

6.2   CONVERSATIONS AND SPEECH ACTS

One of the most fruitful areas in the study of **pragmatics** abilities in PWA is the investigation of conversational abilities and text comprehension. Conversation is the main context for language use and the main linguistic context in which we all learn our mother tongue; it is the most common type of familiar discourse, in which two or more participants take turns speaking and listening, shaping their conversational styles and competence. A conversation is a collaborative act in which participants recognize a common target. What the participants say is determined by the common goal, but what they communicate to each other during this exchange goes beyond the linguistic content of the sentences themselves. Philosophers of language have been interested in modelling how understanding is achieved during a conversation, and how speakers fill the gap between what is explicitly said (the propositional content expressed in a sentence) and what is really meant by the speaker and understood by the listener. According to Grice (1975), a conversation is guided by some fundamental principles. In his seminal studies, Grice has developed a system based on a set of four conversational maxims, which have come to be known as Grice's maxims: the maxim of quality (the demand that the speaker makes a true contribution in the conversation); the maxim of quantity (the contribution should be as informative as required); the maxim of relation (the contribution should be relevant for the current conversation); and the maxim of manner (specifying the contribution should be clear). These maxims are not limited to a specific linguistic act, but they are the root of any collaborative act between humans. Each proposition uttered by speakers during conversation is designed to serve a specific function; it is an action performed through speech. The function each proposition serves is critical to communication, and the listener should be able to recognize which speech act the speaker has performed. The speech act theory (Grice, 1975, 1978; Searle, 1969) describes the acts that can be accomplished by producing a sentence. Examples of speech acts include: informing the listeners, questioning them about a fact, or promising them something. For a speech act to be valid in a conversation, certain conditions must be fulfilled. Every speech act has specific felicity conditions, related to its pragmatics. For example, the act of questioning can be considered felicitous only if the speaker does not know the answer to the question and believes that the listener does. Speech acts are different from the content of the sentence: the speech act identifies the communicative function of a sentence (i.e., the reason why the sentence has been uttered). It is crucial to keep in mind that much of what is understood of an utterance does not come from what is directly said but rather from what is inferred by the listener, hence the crucial role of pragmatics in communication. Grice (1975, 1978) developed the notion of **conversational implicature** to account for this discrepancy between the literal reading of a sentence and the speaker's full meaning. Implicatures are inferences speakers intend the listener to draw from their utterances. Speakers do not spell out each bit of information to which they are referring, and often leave out the most obvious pieces of information for listeners to supply as bridging assumptions. For example, if after this long introduction I pronounce the sentence "This was a short paragraph", it is implicit to the readers that I mean the opposite.

Implicatures are based on a shared knowledge and on a rapid decoding process, which is often performed unconsciously by the listener. The larger the common background between the speaker and the listener, the easier it is to discuss topics without making explicit reference to them. To sum up, for a conversation to run in a productive way, interlocutors utilize some devices—such as common knowledge and the situational and linguistic contexts—that allow the speaker to omit a large part of what he or she wants to say. The listener, on the other hand, must do more than simply take in what the speaker has produced; they must join the bits together of what was meant implicitly. It is clear now that in conversation, here defined as a quite complex sequence of speech acts, the work is distributed between the speaker and the listener. The scope of a conversation is not to tell the truth or to obey to a logic operation; rather, it is more often based on an act of cooperation. What is communicated is not confined to what has been said by the speaker, but incorporates both the environment in which the conversation takes place and also the listener's expectations. The three most important speech acts that have been studied with a severely aphasic patient are: ask a question, state something, and produce the actor to do something. When the clinician is confident that the patient has understood that sentences may be used for different goals, they no longer need to define the nature of the speech act involved (Basso, 2010). This entire long introduction assumes that core aspects of the pragmatic theory, such as the Gricean maxims and the study of speech acts, are remarkably effective tools for implementing conversation therapies based on promoting speech acts. This process may be vastly different if the information to be processed is not embedded in a conversation but is, for example, a discourse reported in a written text.

6.3   Discourse Models in Written Text

Another approach to the investigation of comprehension of complex linguistic units is to investigate the understanding of written text, looking at text variables in people with aphasia. A comprehensive study on text comprehension that has discussed the abilities of a large set of people with different kinds of aphasia reported that syntactic-based variables, such as the number of propositions or syntactic complexity, do not have much of an effect on text comprehension in people with aphasia. In contrast, the type of information integrated in the text is a crucial variable to consider in the investigation of discourse comprehension (Webster et al., 2018). Reading for understanding is a crucial ability in our daily life. Brookshire and colleagues (Brookshire et al., 2014) reported that 68% of people with aphasia experience reading difficulties (using criteria based on reading aloud and not reading comprehension). Despite the reported prevalence of reading difficulties, there is little research about reading for meaning in aphasia compared to reading aloud, particularly for more extended text. It is quite clear that written discourse comprehension is a complex process with both cognitive and linguistic factors known to influence reading ability and reading personal preferences in healthy readers. Factors include individual-level variables such as age (Stine, 1990), social background (e.g., Gleed, 2014), level of education and factors related to the capacity and efficiency of cognitive processes such as attention and memory (Carretti et al., 2009).

In terms of specific linguistic factors, Webster et al. (2018) provides a comprehensive investigation of the influence of text-related variables based on theoretical models of discourse comprehension, adapted to study reading for meaning. The model considered in the study is the construction–integration model proposed by Kintsch (1988). This model involves the construction and integration of material, with discourse organized based on macrostructure and microstructure.

Macrostructure is the coherent organization of the main ideas or themes within the discourse. **Microstructure** is the surface structure of sentences, including the individual words selected and the propositions. Within discourse comprehension, we need to understand the words and sentences, construct the meaning of the text coherent object, and then relate the information to our knowledge of the world. In Kintsch's **construction–integration model**, the first step is the construction phase; this is when the linguistic form is processed, propositions are identified, and inferences are elaborated. The notion of proposition is crucial for this first phase. A proposition is "the smallest unit of knowledge that can stand alone; it has defined as a unit that has a truth value – that is, a proposition can be either true or false." During the scanning of a text, propositions are extracted from the overall text and organized according to the topics they share. For example, the main ideas within the text are repeated across propositions and form a macrostructure (main idea). Details related to the main ideas are not repeated and form the microstructure (main details). In coherent text, the details of a text must be linked to one another and to the main idea. The second stage of Kintsch's model that follows the construction phase is the integration phase, where information is integrated into a coherent entity with no ambiguous or incorrect inference. This involves a series of processes, including going back to information that has already been specified, and linking the propositions that are already built and stored in episodic memory. The structure of the meaning of the full text has then to be integrated with the general knowledge of the world. Another crucial aspect of the text analysis is related to the information that is not openly written in the text but may need to be inferred. In Fig. 6.1, we have reported one example of a short story from Webster et al. (2018)'s study and the questions related to the comprehension of the paragraph (see Table 6.1). Questions were presented in a multiple-choice format, with a target answer and two possible distractors.

Data from this study report that inferential meaning (both main ideas - implied and detail - implied) are the most vulnerable aspects in

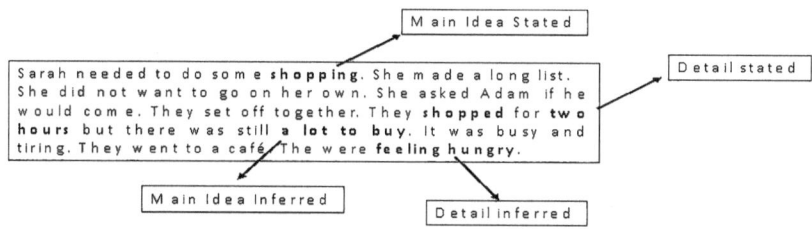

Fig. 6.1 A paragraph adopted in Webster et al.'s (2018) reading study with discourse factors affecting reading for understandings

Table 6.1 Set of questions and multiple-choice answers with target and distractors adopted for comprehension of the paragraph in Fig. 6.1, from Webster et al. (2018)

	Questions	TARGET	DISTRACTOR 1	DISTRACTOR 2
MIS	Sarah and Adam went	shopping	for a walk	to the cinema
DS	They shopped	for two hours	all morning	for four hours
DI	They stopped to get	a meal	a drink	more money
MII	Sarah needed to buy	many things	a few things	a present

MIS main idea stated, *DS* detail stated, *DI* Detail implied, *MII* main idea implied

both healthy controls and, even more so, in PWA, with no other effects related to the length of the paragraph or the grammatical complexity. Inferential processing is defined as the derivation of additional knowledge from facts already known; this might involve going beyond the literal meaning of a passage to gain more coherence or to get an extra knowledge of the facts.

There are several kinds of inferences in language: logical, bridging, and elaborative. Logical inference arises from the links between the word meaning. Bridging inferences link the most current information to some information stated in a previous part of the text (see box below). Elaborative inferences are made when we extend what is in the text using world knowledge. Future studies should evaluate in more detail the nature of the inferential process costs in people with aphasia and whether cognitive factors are at the core of vulnerable inferential processing or more specific pragmatic factors.

Inferential Processing: Filling the Dots

Inferential processing is defined as the extra operation of additional knowledge from facts already known; this might involve going beyond the literal meaning of a passage/discourse to gain more coherence or to get an extra knowledge of the facts. There are several kinds of inferential processing based on the cognitive operation required to the speaker: logical, bridging, and elaborative.

Logical inference arises from the links between the semantics of the word, and its meaning. There are different forms of logical inferences. One example is the syllogism: "All meat comes from animals. All beef is meat. Therefore, all beef comes from animals." Incorrect logical inferences are called fallacy. Cognitive psychologists have documented many **cognitive biases** in human reasoning that favor incorrect reasoning, for example in relation to social stereotypes.

Bridging inferences link the most recent information to some information stated in a previous part of the text. One example is: "The bridge collapsed. The wood was rotten." The inference connects the word bridge and the word wood to the event described in the sentence: "The bridge collapsed because the wood of the bridge was rotten." This is a very powerful inferential mechanism that requires cognitive resources.

Elaborative inferences are made when we extend what is in the text using world knowledge. An example is: "The fridge is full of food. Someone has gone for a large shopping."

Future studies should evaluate in more detail the nature of the inferential process in people with aphasia and if cognitive factors are at the core of vulnerable inferential processing (Wright & Newhoff, 2004).

6.4   COHERENCE IN APHASIC DISCOURSE

The definition of main ideas and details as the core components of discourse emphasizes the importance of information processing, more than linguistic factors, within a text. Both main ideas and details must be linked and integrated in order for a text to be coherent. The coherence of a text is a fundamental aspect, meaning not only that a text can be read accurately, but also that clear cues are given for integrating sentences into other components, such as long-term memory and encyclopaedic knowledge (Haarmann et al., 1997). A very well-structured and coherent text may compensate for cognitive limitations in memory and for slow processing. If paragraphs in a text do not follow a logical and coherent order it takes longer for a reader to understand and to read, with some problems for people with language disorders. Some studies reported discourse coherence to be impaired in aphasia; others found it to be well preserved. This set of conflicting findings could be attributed to different frameworks and definitions used by researchers. In a recent study, coherence in people with aphasia was addressed in a richer paradigm and operationalized through the combination of four aspects: informativeness, clarity, connectedness, and understandability (Linnik et al., 2022). Coherence has been defined as a property of both internal links at discourse level but also the quality of language in use, co-constructed by a speaker and the listener or reader. The main findings of the study indicated that a well-formed discourse structure was especially important for two aspects of coherence—informativeness and understandability. This suggests that a shared pragmatic knowledge could boost coherence, as it helps interlocutors to compensate for language deficits.

6.5   Assessment of Pragmatics in Aphasia

The view supported by the neoclassical notion of aphasia as a unitary disorder is based on the idea that language in people with aphasia is not lost but inaccessible. The pragmatic approach to language treatment is derived from the application of pragmatic theories to aphasia therapy. In general, it puts the emphasis on communication and its related skills more than specific components of language. The interest in conversational abilities and communication in aphasia began in the late 1960s and early 1970s, when the focus of treatment moved from the specific disorder to the functional use of language in more naturalistic contexts, for example in spontaneous conversations. Based on the findings that pragmatic and communication abilities are well preserved in people with aphasia, and on a more general therapy target based on improving communication, the assessment of pragmatic aspects became more relevant for the design of a therapeutic program (Basso, 2010). A first evaluation tool of pragmatic abilities, the Functional Communication Profile (FCP), was developed by M.T. Sarno in 1969, and later the Communicative Abilities in Daily Living (CADL) was published and revised in 1999 (CADL-2; Holland et al., 1999). The CADL-2 framework is adapted from Searle's theory of speech acts (Searle, 1969) and targets communication activities that occur in daily life, creating the relevant scenario for the activity. It tests specific aspects of communication: social communication, requesting information, and correcting misinterpretation with no emphasis of a specific modality or linguistic aspects. Any media including gestures are accepted. Pragmatic tests are not developed for replacing more traditional assessments for aphasia, such as, for instance, the Boston Diagnostic Assessment Examination (BDAE; Goodglass & Kaplan, 1982) or the Western Aphasia Battery (WAB; Kertesz, 1982). Instead, these tests supplement the standard aphasia assessments by adding a more diverse aspect of language which is usually not included in standard aphasia batteries. The main target of pragmatic interventions is broader than that of therapies directed to remediate a language module or a specific language operation. The overall approach of the pragmatics intervention is less prescriptive and based on favoring communicative strategies allowing the aphasic individual to interact more easily with others, using any mode of communication and with the direct involvement of the patient environment. Treatments based on pragmatics include both the Supporting Conversation for Adults with Aphasia (SCA; Kagan, 1998) and Conversational Coaching (Hopper et al., 2002).

Conversational Coaching involves teaching individuals with aphasia and their carers the use of a set of communication strategies, such as clarification, requesting circumlocution, drawing, verifying comprehension, writing, and gesturing—all in addition to, or in substitution of, speech. It usually starts by observing the conversational strategies which the individual is adopting during communication with family and careers. It works with pre-recorded materials integrated into a system of training; if the content of this new material is understood by the person with aphasia, the carer is invited to join the session for the person with aphasia in order to attempt to communicate the story. Most of the clinician interventions are directed to coach the person with aphasia to listen carefully and to instruct the individual without aphasia to frequently ask for clarification. In a recent study involving two dyads (Hopper et al., 2002), significant training effects were found after 10 sessions in the number of main concepts successfully communicated. Similar positive communication outcomes have been reported following SCA (Kagan, 1998), based on a similar assumption that people with aphasia know more than they are able to express in verbal speech.

6.6   Application and Therapeutic Approaches

Current methods for targeting pragmatic therapy can be divided into two main categories. The first category includes utterance-focused aphasia test batteries, which concentrate on isolated verbal expression skills, such as naming objects, describing scenes, or repeating words and sentences, without considering their communicative purpose. The second category consists of dialogue-sensitive diagnostic tools in SLT, which aim to assess communication skills in everyday contexts through role-playing or questionnaires, with input from clinicians and family members. Aligned with the view that language emerges from social interaction, linguistic-pragmatic theory suggests that dialogue-sensitive diagnostic tools address a broader range of communicative aspects than utterance-centred methods. For instance, verbal requests differ from object naming in that they involve a more complex action–sequence structure, shared "common ground," and an understanding of the conversation partner's assumptions and intentions (Theory of Mind).

There are few studies on treatment methods targeting the reading of paragraphs and connected text which aim to improve reading comprehension. People with aphasia usually report a positive feeling when they try to understand information within a paragraph, despite significant difficulties with the comprehension of single words and sentences. The main idea is to challenge the simplistic assumption (held both by people with aphasia and by clinicians) that texts are harder than shorter sentences and that difficulty increases with increasing length of paragraph. Within a well-written and coherent paragraph, redundancy and repetition of information is an asset to support comprehension. This does not detract from a potential influence of confidence in ability; in this study readers began with (very) short paragraphs, with these increasing over time; this may have contributed to their perception of ability and willingness to attempt the task (Webster et al., 2013).

People with aphasia were better able to understand main ideas than details and stated than inferred information. This can be considered further in terms of the type of comprehension required to understand genres of text, and this could be utilized within intervention. For certain genres of text, facilitating understanding of those main ideas could be most beneficial and for other types of text, strategies to ensure comprehension of relevant detail could be more helpful. The important finding that establishing meaning over time was particularly difficult for people with aphasia also requires further consideration, given the relevance of this for many reading activities.

6.7   Summary

Reading paragraphs as well as taking part in conversations are important everyday activities which play a key role in participation in social and work domains for many individuals. Reading comprehension is impaired for many people with aphasia, but not necessarily all. We need to consider the complexities of reading, of different genres, the purpose of reading, individual reading ability and preferences and relationships between different reading skills. Information about discourse comprehension in people with aphasia has come from studies of spoken comprehension, providing some potential indicators of factors affecting written discourse. It has been suggested that the redundancy and context present in discourse can compensate for lexical and grammatical difficulties at both word and sentence level (Brookshire & Nicholas, 1984). Meteyard et al. (2015) investigated inferential comprehension in four people with chronic aphasia who reported having adequate written single word and sentence comprehension but difficulties in reading texts. They investigated inferential comprehension by comparing factual versus inferential reading on the MCLA and using a specifically designed inference task contrasting understanding of local and global inferences. They define local inferences as those requiring interpretation based on links between successive words and sentences and global inferences as those needing integration of world knowledge (Meteyard et al., 2015). Varied patterns of reading comprehension difficulties were seen across the four participants, with different patterns of retained and impaired performance across factual and inferential reading and the understanding of local and global inferences.

6.8   Discussion Topics

1. Speech acts have been studied with severely aphasic patients. Define two or three speech acts and how they can be promoted in conversation therapies.
2. Discuss the inferential processing that occurs during a conversation with examples relevant for speakers with aphasia.
3. Reading for understanding is a core ability for reaching the complex meaning of a text. Define, with some examples, the meaning of the terms microstructural and macrostructural factors.
4. Describe the main kind of information involved in discourse comprehension according to the construction–integration model proposed by Kintsch (1988). What is the evidence collected for speakers with aphasia?

5. Present pragmatic intervention models and describe what they target. Why is it important to integrate pragmatic evaluation to more standard assessments?
6. Define what text coherence is by discussing research on aphasia.

REFERENCES

Basso, A. (2010). "Natural" conversation: A treatment for severe aphasia. *Aphasiology, 24*(4), 466–479.

Brookshire, C. E., Wilson, J. P., Nadeau, S. E., Gonzalez Rothi, L. J., & Kendall, D. L. (2014). Frequency, nature, and predictors of alexia in a convenience sample of individuals with chronic aphasia. *Aphasiology, 28*(12), 1464–1480.

Brookshire, R. H., & Nicholas, L. E. (1984). Comprehension of directly and indirectly stated main ideas and details in discourse by brain-damaged and non-brain-damaged listeners. *Brain and Language, 21*(1), 21–36.

Carretti, B., Borella, E., Cornoldi, C., & De Beni, R. (2009). Role of working memory in explaining the performance of individuals with specific reading comprehension difficulties: A meta-analysis. *Learning and Individual Differences, 19*(2), 246–251.

Gleed, A. (2014). Booktrust reading habits survey 2013: A national survey of reading habits and attitudes to books amongst adults in England: Retrieved from the Booktrust website. http://www.booktrust.org.uk

Goodglass, H., & Kaplan, E. (1982). *The assessment of aphasia and related disorders* (2nd ed.). Lea & Febiger.

Grice, H. P. (1975). Logic and conversation. In P. Cole & G. Morgan (Eds.), *Speech acts: Syntax and semantics* (Vol. 3, pp. 199–219). Academic Press.

Grice, H. P. (1978). Some further notes on logic and conversation. In P. Cole & J. Morgan (Eds.), *Syntax and semantics* (Vol. 9, pp. 113–128). Academic Press.

Haarmann, H. J., Just, M. A., & Carpenter, P. A. (1997). Aphasic sentence comprehension as a resource deficit: A computational approach. *Brain and Language, 59*(1), 76–120.

Happé, F., Brownell, H., & Winner, E. (1999). Acquired 'theory of mind' impairments following stroke. *Cognition, 70*, 211–240.

Holland, A. L., Frattali, C., & Fromm, D. (1999). *Communicative activities of daily living (CADL-2)*. Pro-Ed.

Hopper, T., Holland, A. L., & Rewega, M. (2002). Conversational coaching: Treatment outcomes and future directions. *Aphasiology, 16*, 745–761.

Kagan, A. (1998). Supported conversation for adults with aphasia: Methods and resources for training conversation partners. *Aphasiology, 12*, 816–829.

Kertesz, A. (1982). *The Western Aphasia Battery*. Grune & Stratton.

Kertesz, A. (1988). Cognitive function in severe aphasia. In L. Weiskrantz (Ed.), *Thought without language* (pp. 451–463). Oxford University Press.

Kintsch, W. (1988). The role of knowledge in discourse comprehension: A construction–integration model. *Psychological Review, 95*(2), 163–182.

Linnik, A., Bastiaanse, R., Stede, M., & Khudyakova, M. (2022). Linguistic mechanisms of coherence in aphasic and non-aphasic discourse. *Aphasiology, 36*(2), 123–146.

Meteyard, L., Bruce, C., Edmundson, A., & Oakhill, J. (2015). Profiling text comprehension impairments in aphasia. *Aphasiology, 29*(1), 1–28.

Osman, D. M., Shohdi, S., & Aziz, A. A. (2011). Pragmatic difficulties in children with specific language impairment. *International Journal of Pediatric Otorhinolaryngology, 75*(2), 171–176. https://doi.org/10.1016/j.ijporl.2010.10.028

Rossi, L., Garraffa, M., & Surian, L. (2013). Do children with specific language impairment (SLI) have a deficit in detecting violations of Gricean maxims? *Psicologia clinica dello sviluppo, Rivista quadrimestrale, 1*(2013), 135–146. https://doi.org/10.1449/73830

Sarno, M. T. (1969). *Functional communication profile: A manual of directions.* Rehabilitation Monograph 42. NYU Medical Center.

Searle, J. R. (1969). *Speech acts.* Cambridge University Press.

Siegal, M., Valery, R., & Want, S. (2001). Mind over grammar: Reasoning in aphasia and development. *Trends in Cognitive Sciences, 5*(7), 296–301.

Stine, E. A. L. (1990). 11 the way Reading and listening work: A tutorial review of discourse processing and aging. *Advances in Psychology, 72*, 301–327.

Varley, R., & Siegal, M. (2000). Evidence for cognition without grammar from causal reasoning and 'theory of mind' in an agrammatic aphasic patient. *Current Biology, 10*, 723–726.

Webster, J., Morris, J., Connor, C., Horner, R., McCormac, C., & Potts, A. (2013). Text level reading comprehension in aphasia: What do we know about therapy and what do we need to know? *Aphasiology, 27*(11), 1362–1380.

Webster, J., Morris, J., Howard, D., & Garraffa, M. (2018). Reading for meaning: What influences paragraph understanding in aphasia? *American Journal of Speech-Language Pathology, 27*, 423–437. https://doi.org/10.1044/2017_AJSLP-16-0213

Wright, H. H., & Newhoff, M. (2004). Inference revision processing in adults with and without aphasia. *Brain & Language, 3*, 450–463. https://doi.org/10.1016/S0093-934X(03)00469-3

CHAPTER 7

Current Topics in Linguistics and Aphasia

Abstracts This final chapter will incorporate insights about aphasiology not only from theoretical linguistics, but also from other aspects of the language sciences, such as bilingual aphasia, sociolinguistics, neurolinguistics and medical humanities with the intention of opening a richer dialogue between aphasiology and the language sciences. Some open questions will be presented, such as the specificity of the linguistic disorders for the aphasia syndromes compared to other language disorders in adulthood and the general issue about aphasia classifications in group studies.

It will also address how linguistics can contribute to a more detailed classification of the language disorder in aphasia if combined with modern technologies applied to therapies such as brain stimulations. The chapter ends with some discussion topics on the effect of global demographic changes, such as the increase of multilingualism, that need to be considered in research and practice of acquired language disorders.

Keywords Multimodal therapy • Language non-specific deficit • Multidimensional deficit • Bilingual aphasia

M. Garraffa, G. Smith, *Linguistic Theory for Aphasia*,
https://doi.org/10.1007/978-3-031-77134-7_7

7.1   A Linguistic-Based Approach to Aphasia: Some Considerations

The approach advocated in this book emphasizes a linguistic-based method for investigating language in individuals with aphasia, which has significant methodological implications. Traditional patient–group research, categorized by classical syndrome types, has been criticized for not providing a comprehensive understanding of language deficits in aphasia, echoing earlier findings from the 1980s (Caramazza & Martin, 1983). This syndrome-based approach lacks clarity in defining language impairments and does not align well with comprehensive linguistics investigations of the language of a person with aphasia within the framework presented in this book. Instead, the syndrome-based approach often serves practical purposes such as study design efficiency and clinical record organization rather than focusing on the core language properties of the disorder.

For example, many group studies distinguishing between non-fluent and fluent aphasia may not be sufficient for developing a robust language model, as non-fluent aphasia encompasses diverse underlying factors and cannot be considered a factor to create homogenous groups (see, for example, Aziz et al., 2024 for a study on sentence comprehension in fluent and non-fluent aphasia). A more effective approach involves detailed descriptions of linguistic functions across languages and linguistic domains within individual speakers to avoid misclassification of the language disorder into non-linguistics categories based on classifications not entirely justified by the language system.

Consequently, if the aim is to address fundamental language disorder issues, patient–group research based solely on classical syndrome types may not be appropriate. However, this doesn't imply that all patient–group research is methodologically unacceptable. Rather, it underscores the need for a clear linguistic framework to derive insights from both single and group patient studies.

Methodological and theoretical precautions are essential for patient–group research. Patients should be grouped based on linguistically motivated dimensions, thereby ensuring homogeneity regarding the impaired language components. Empirical support for these dimensions should come from a comprehensive linguistic analysis of each patient's performance across various tasks, confirming that the group-defining behavior reflects consistent impairment in the targeted language component. This approach, termed the "group/case study approach," involves studying a group of patients extensively while investigating individual differences (Caramazza & Martin, 1983), thus avoiding that patients whose source of the language disorder is different be grouped together and also to group patients with a different neurological diagnosis into a similar linguistic group. This point will be expanded in the next section, where language disorders such as the one reported in people with aphasia in other adult populations will be discussed.

7.2 LINGUISTIC DISORDERS ACROSS THE ADULT POPULATION

In this volume, we have discussed how the linguistic disorder presents itself in adults following a neurological event in the brain. For many years, the language of aphasic patients was considered the specific by-product of an abrupt interruption of access to linguistic resources in a mature language system, and consequently inherently different from other atypical linguistic profiles. However, this notion has been challenged by results in recent decades showing similarities between the language of aphasic patients and that of other, non-acquired conditions affecting language. This is the case, for example, for dementia. Dementia is an umbrella term which groups together different degenerative disorders, including Alzheimer's disease (AD), Parkinson's disease (PD), and frontotemporal dementia (FTD). A subtype of frontotemporal dementia, known as Primary Progressive Aphasia (PPA), is specifically identified for its effects on language. These include impairments in the lexical-semantic domain (the semantic variant, svPPA), agrammatism (non-fluent/agrammatic variant, nfvPPA), and more (Montembeault et al., 2018). It is interesting to note that in a recent study on nfvPPA comparing two groups of patients speaking respectively English and Italian, nfvPPA-affected English speakers showed greater motor speech impairment than nfvPPA-affected Italian speakers, despite higher levels of education and comparable disease severity and atrophy changes. On the other hand, greater grammatical impairment was reported in nfvPPA-Italian compared to the English group. This study illustrates the need to consider the effect of the individual's spoken language for a precise schematization of the phenotype and clinical presentation of PPA variants, suggesting that knowledge of the linguistics and the pattern of use of it is essential to evaluate nfvPPA (Canu et al., 2020).

Disorders of language that resemble those described in acquired aphasia have been found across the board in dementia-type disorders. Impairments in the lexical-semantic domain, which are typical of anomia, have been addressed systematically, for example noun and verb naming (Cappa et al., 1998; Almor et al., 2009). Although investigated less frequently, findings of morphosyntactic disorders attested in agrammatic aphasia have also been replicated in AD, including verb-related morphosyntactic production (Fyndanis et al., 2013).

The similarities in the linguistic profiles of atypical speakers across conditions do not limit themselves to abnormal brain injury or decay, but also extend to another category of speakers, namely those affected by neurodevelopmental disorders (NDDs). A group of disorders with onset in childhood, NNDs include autism spectrum disorders (ASD), attention-deficit/hyperactivity disorders (ADHD), intellectual disabilities (ID), communication disorders (dyslexia, specific language disorder, and others), and more. Much like with PPA and dementia, a disorder of language is at the basis of the symptomatology of a communication disorder, but it is found across all NDDs in both children and adults (Smith et al., 2023). For example, simpler spontaneous productions in terms of grammatical structures used and number of verbs compared to controls was found in ID and ASD (Loveall et al., 2019; Altman et al., 2022; Geelhand et al., 2021).

These findings question the idea that language disorders reported in adults may be specific to language-based conditions such as aphasia and communication disorders. A new scenario seems more plausible with communalities of language features impaired across conditions based on linguistics predictions.

7.3   Multilingualism and Aphasia

Multilingualism may be defined as using more than one language in everyday life (Garraffa et al., 2023). In aphasia, multilingualism has implications for diagnosis and rehabilitation. A crucial issue posed in diagnosing the level of post-stroke language abilities in bilingual speakers with aphasia is how to reliably determine pre-stroke language abilities. This is problematic in monolinguals too, but particularly so in multilingual patients, who typically have different proficiency levels in different language domains for each language and often across language modalities (see Aziz et al., 2020, 2024 for studies on colloquial Malay). The outcomes of aphasia in multilingual individuals are determined not just by factors which are critical in monolinguals, such as level of education and literacy, but also by other factors such as pre-stroke language abilities and the age of acquisition of each language (Lerman et al., 2020).

To assess these factors as best as possible, some specific tools have been developed, including the Bilingual Aphasia Test (BAT; Paradis & Libben, 2014) and the Bilingual Aphasia Summary form (Kohnert, 2013). The BAT, for instance, is a useful tool available online which has been translated and adapted into over 60 languages and is composed of a questionnaire on language use and a series of linguistic assessments for each language. An additional assessment of specific language pairs, for example English–Spanish or English–Arabic, is available for several languages, and it contains tasks such as translation from language A to language B and from language B to language A. As with any self-reported questionnaire, however, there still is an issue of reliability.

Recovery patterns across the different languages can see different outcomes among multilingual speakers and can be either parallel or selective. In parallel recovery patterns, languages are affected similarly by the stroke. In contrast, in selective patterns, one language, typically the one acquired first (Kuzmina et al., 2019), is selectively more preserved than another. Several are the topics that are being addressed in relation to the asymmetry of recovery, including the role of executive control in preserving language(s) (Mooijman et al., 2022), whether some aspects of language show more of an asymmetry than others (for example, lexical semantic access), and whether multilingualism constitutes an overall advantage in cognitive reserve in aphasia (Peñaloza et al., 2020).

The existing body of literature on aphasia falls short of representing the diverse linguistic landscape of the world, in terms of both linguistic typology and the sheer number of speakers. This prevalent bias towards English and other Western European languages not only restricts the global relevance of clinical insights, especially in aphasia therapy, but also challenges the universality of theoretical frameworks derived from observations primarily made in a handful of closely related languages. Hence, it is imperative to prioritize the development of a more cross-linguistic approach to aphasia in future research endeavors. By broadening our understanding across different languages, we can enhance the effectiveness of therapeutic interventions and ensure inclusivity in addressing this complex neurological condition on a global scale (Beveridge & Bak, 2011).

7.4   Sociolinguistics in the Aphasic Clinic

As stated in the previous section, most speakers in the world can communicate in more than one language. Logically, bilingual aphasia is ordinary—an not an extraordinary—feature, which is often neglected in the clinic. There are several challenges associated to assessing a bilingual speaker that go beyond language proper, but SLTs, being trained in linguistics, are always the preferred interlocutors for a language assessment in any of the languages spoken by the patient. A line of research on bilingual speakers with aphasia has addressed the question of whether bilingualism, a known protective factor on neural degeneration, can have a protective effect from the incidence of a stroke, and/or its severity. Preliminary research is reporting encouraging data about learning additional languages as a protective factor both before and after an acquired brain injury (Dekhtyar et al., 2020). The main purpose of this research is to record that being bilingual is not actually affecting your brain in a negative way. Indeed, some studies are reporting a possible correlation whereby although bilingual speakers are at equal risk as monolinguals of developing aphasia after a stroke, their aphasia is likely to be less severe, a characteristic that has important implications on recovery patterns and quality of life after a stroke (Paplikar et al., 2019).

Additional research on bilingual aphasia can also have an impact on speech and language therapy. More awareness about the properties of different languages can lead to the development of better rehabilitation protocols and intervention in language disorders (Crowley et al., 2015). Learning about (socio)linguistic issues during SLT training is rare in aphasia centers and in centers with a high number of patients from ethnic minorities; there are challenges among therapists whose language properties are very different from their patients (e.g., Charity Hudley et al., 2018). Unfortunately, the disparities in linguistic varieties may lead to misdiagnoses in patients who do not speak the same variety as those who are assessing their language disorder. To improve health service and reduce health inequality, more SLTs are needed who can speak and use more than one language, better reflect their patient populations, and can apply sociolinguistic understanding of language variation in their assessment and intervention efforts.

7.5   PATIENT-CENTERED APPROACH: BRAIN STIMULATION AND LANGUAGE MODELS

Modern aphasia rehabilitation principles advocate for a patient-centric approach, beginning with a comprehensive assessment of language impairments and subsequently tailoring rehabilitation techniques to align with the identified language profile. Some therapeutic frameworks incorporate non-invasive brain stimulation methods, such as repetitive transcranial magnetic stimulation (TMS), transcranial direct current stimulation (tDCS), or epidural electrical stimulation (EES), as detailed in Bhattacharya et al. (2022).

The promising outcomes yielded by these plasticity-induced techniques, coupled with minimal contraindications, render them highly desirable. However, it remains imperative to establish safety protocols to maximize their effectiveness across all stages of post-stroke aphasia management (Holland & Crinion, 2012). These stimulation methods aim to enhance language performance by either increasing the total amount of learning achieved, thereby reaching a higher performance level, or accelerating the rate at which learning occurs, achieving the same maximum performance level as standard therapy but in a shorter timeframe, and thus requiring fewer hours of behavioral therapy.

Tasks conducted during non-invasive brain stimulations encompass verbal fluency (Iyer et al., 2005), picture naming (Fertonani et al., 2010; Sparing et al., 2007), proper name retrieval (Ross et al., 2010), nonword–picture matching (Fiori et al., 2011), and a diverse array of tDCS protocols and stimulation sites. Current evidence suggests that the stimulation applied to the left hemisphere language cortices, compared to sham (no stimulation), significantly enhances normal language performance in terms of reaction time or accuracy. This is a fresh territory for aphasia therapy in which linguistics protocols can provide a well-defined set of predictions and more detailed item analyses, creating convergence systems between linguistics and neuroscience.

7.6   NARRATIVE MEDICINE: COMMUNICATION WITH PEOPLE WITH APHASIA

Language serves as more than just a medical symptom across various linguistic domains; it is a vital resource in clinical practice, particularly as cognitive disorders become more prevalent in the aging global population. Conversations between patients with aphasia and clinicians offer valuable insights into the challenges faced in these interactions, highlighting the need for further research in narrative medicine (see Garraffa & Mazzaggio 2025, for an introduction to Pragmatics in Health Care Practice). Ineffective communication ranks among the leading causes of sentinel events in healthcare, with individuals with communication disabilities at higher risk of preventable adverse events in hospitals (Lamborn et al., 2024). Studies show that approximately 51% of aphasia patients encounter difficulties in comprehending or expressing treatment-related information during hospitalization (O'Halloran et al., 2012). For instance, the Inpatient Functional Communication Interview (IFCI) offers SLTs an interview tool to assess the communication support needs of individual patients in hospital settings and provides three audit tools for the multidisciplinary team to evaluate communication supports within the hospital system (O'Halloran et al., 2024). This exemplifies an environment-level assessment emphasizing communication as fundamental to the care of aphasia patients.

Research observing conversations between stroke patients and nurses revealed limited opportunities for aphasia patients to communicate with nurses compared to those without speech impairments (Hersh et al., 2016). Patients with communication difficulties are over six times more likely to experience patient safety incidents than general patients (Bartlett et al., 2008). Among medical staff, nurses have the most significant communication role with aphasia patients, significantly impacting patient care (Hersh et al., 2016).

Stroke, the primary cause of aphasia, necessitates collaborative communication among various healthcare members, including doctors, nurses, therapists, and caregivers. Participants emphasized the importance of systems facilitating information sharing about patients' language issues among healthcare providers to enhance communication with aphasic patients (Hur & Kang, 2022). They expressed a desire for education on effective communication methods, including devices, media, and universally recognized agreements. Nurses with extensive experience in communicating with aphasic patients demonstrated better communication skills, drawing from their firsthand experiences in caring for patients with communication disorders (O'Halloran et al., 2012; Cheba et al., 2014). However, they often lacked formal training in effective communication strategies and in the specific aspects of language more often impaired in people with aphasia.

7.7   Summary

In this chapter we have very briefly identified some topics that the current research in aphasiology is facing in relation to language abilities. Innovation in the available technology, as in the case of non-invasive brain stimulation is now a possible scenario to accelerate or compensate for long hours of speech therapy. In this approach a detailed language profile is essentially paired with a therapeutical protocol based on incremental targets in convergence with linguistics. It is also necessary to consider that individuals in the contemporary society are more dynamic and this is mirrored in an increase of bilingual speakers, but unfortunately with a lack of representation of several natural languages in research and in the assessment tools available. All these components, together with a lack of representation of the syndrome-based model in language disorders, are in support of the idea that linguistics is now an essential element to better understand the level and the component damaged but also to design a specific and effective protocol for innovative rehabilitation plans.

7.8   Discussion Topics

1. In this chapter, we have discussed the distinctions between group and individual studies in aphasia. Discuss which factors are necessary for a good design in a group study. Provide an application of these factors by proposing a study design.
2. Bilingualism is the norm in many countries. Discuss the consequences of bilingualism in aphasiology by reporting evidence from research on multilingual aphasia.
3. Explain the communalities of language disorders in adults between acquired, developmental, and degenerative disorders.
4. What should be the role of speech and language therapists in bilingual aphasia? And in working with speakers of minority languages?
5. Why is important to collect a detailed language profile of a bilingual aphasic speaker? Provide examples from case studies supported with research evidence.
6. Brain stimulation is one of the new frontiers of language therapy. Discuss the role of linguistics theory in this new therapeutical horizon and consequences for the SLT's job.

REFERENCES

Almor, A., Aronoff, J. M., MacDonald, M. C., Gonnerman, L. M., Kempler, D., Hintiryan, H., Hayes, U. L., Arunachalam, S., & Andersen, E. S. (2009). A common mechanism in verb and noun naming deficits in Alzheimer's patients. *Brain and Language, 111*(1), 8–19.

Altman, C., Avraham, I., Meirovich, S. S., & Lifshitz, H. (2022). How do students with intellectual disabilities tell stories? An investigation of narrative macrostructure and microstructure. *Journal of Applied Research in Intellectual Disabilities, 35*(5), 1119–1130.

Aziz, M. A., Razak, R., & Garraffa, M. (2020). Targeting complex orthography in the treatment of bilingual dysgraphia: A case of a Malay/English speaker with conduction aphasia. *Behavioural Science, 10*(7), 109–122.

Aziz, M. A. A., Smith, G., Alisaputri, M. L., Abdul Hamid, B., & Garraffa, M. (2024). S Sentence comprehension in Malay-speaking adults with aphasia: The role of affix integration. *Aphasiology*. Special issue on Across countries, cultures and languages: Assessing aphasia in diverse clinical populations. https://doi.org/10.1080/02687038.2024.2406577.

Bartlett, G., Blais, R., Tamblyn, R., Clermont, R. J., & MacGibbon, B. (2008). Impact of patient communication problems on the risk of preventable adverse events in acute care settings. *Cmaj, 178*(12), 1555–1562.

Beveridge, M. E. L., & Bak, T. H. (2011). The languages of aphasia research: Bias and diversity. *Aphasiology, 25*(12), 1451–1468. https://doi.org/10.108 0/02687038.2011.624165

Bhattacharya, A., Mrudula, K., Sreepada, S. S., Sathyaprabha, T. N., Pal, P. K., Chen, R., & Udupa, K. (2022). An overview of non-invasive brain stimulation: Basic principles and clinical applications. *Can J Neurol Science, 49*(4), 479–492. https://doi.org/10.1017/cjn.2021.158

Canu, E., Agosta, F., Battistella, G., et al. (2020). Speech production differences in English and Italian speakers with non-fluent variant PPA. *Neurology, 94*(10), e1062–e1072.

Cappa, S. F., Binetti, G., Pezzini, A., Padovani, A., Rozzini, L., & Trabucchi, M. (1998). Object and action naming in Alzheimer's disease and frontotemporal dementia. *Neurology, 50*(2), 351–355. https://doi.org/10.1212/WNL.50.2.351

Caramazza, A., & Martin, R. (1983). Theoretical and methodological issues in the study of aphasia. In J. B. Hellige (Ed.), *Cerebral hemisphere asymmetry: Method, theory and application*. Praeger Scientific Publishers.

Charity Hudley, A. H., Mallinson, C., Sudler, K., & Fama, M. (2018). The sociolinguistically trained speech-language pathologist: Using knowledge of African American English to aid and empower African American clientele. *Perspectives of the ASHA Special Interest Groups, 3*(1), 118–131.

Cheba, M., Żuralska, R., & Skrzypek-Czerko, M. (2014). Difficulties related to the communication with the patient with aphasia according to the nursing staff. *Pielęgniarstwo Neurologiczne i Neurochirurgiczne, 3*(2), 75–80.

Crowley, C. J., Guest, K., & Sudler, K. (2015). Cultural competence needed to distinguish disorder from difference: Beyond Kumbaya. Perspectives on Communication Disorders and Sciences in Culturally and Linguistically Diverse (CLD) *Populations, 22*(2), 64–76.

Dekhtyar, M., Kiran, S., & Gray, T. (2020). Is bilingualism protective for adults with aphasia? *Neuropsychologia, 139,* 107355.

Fertonani, A., Rosini, S., Cotelli, M., Rossini, P. M., & Miniussi, C. (2010). Naming facilitation induced by transcranial direct current stimulation. *Behavioural Brain Research, 208*(2), 311–318.

Fiori, V., Coccia, M., Marinelli, C. V., Vecchi, V., Bonifazi, S., Ceravolo, M. G., Provinciali, L., Tomaiuolo, F., & Marangolo, P. (2011). Transcranial direct current stimulation improves word retrieval in healthy and nonfluent aphasic subjects. *Journal of Cognitive Neuroscience, 23*(9), 2309–2323.

Fyndanis,V.,Manouilidou,C.,Koufou,E.,Karampekios,S.,&Tsapakis,E.M.(2013). Agrammatic patterns in Alzheimer's disease: Evidence from tense, agreement, and aspect. *Aphasiology, 27,* 178–200. https://doi.org/10.1080/0268703 8.2012.705814

Garraffa, M., & Mazzaggio, G. (2025). *Pragmatics in the health sciences.* Cambridge University Press.

Garraffa, M., Sorace, A., & Vender, M. (2023). *Bilingualism matters: Language learning across the lifespan.* Cambridge University Press.

Geelhand, P., Papastamou, F., & Kissine, M. (2021). How do autistic adults use syntactic and prosodic cues to manage spoken discourse? *Clinical Linguistics & Phonetics, 35*(12), 1184–1209.

Hersh, D., Godecke, E., Armstrong, E., Ciccone, N., & Bernhardt, J. (2016). "Ward talk:" Nurses' interaction with people with and without aphasia in the very early period poststroke. *Aphasiology, 30*(5), 609–628.

Holland, R., & Crinion, J. (2012). Can tDCS enhance treatment of aphasia after stroke? *Aphasiology, 26*(9), 1169–1191.

Hur, Y., & Kang, Y. (2022). Nurses' experiences of communicating with patients with aphasia. *Nursing Open, 9*(1), 714–720. https://doi.org/10.1002/nop2.1124

Iyer, M. B., Mattu, U., Grafman, J., Lomarev, M., Sato, S., & Wassermann, E. M. (2005). Safety and cognitive effect of frontal DC brain polarization in healthy individuals. *Neurology, 64*(5), 872–875.

Kohnert, K. (2013). *Language disorders in bilingual children and adults* (2nd ed.). Plural.

Kuzmina, E., Goral, M., Norvik, M., & Weekes, B. S. (2019). What influences language impairment in bilingual aphasia? *A meta-analytic review. Frontiers in psychology, 10,* 445.

Lamborn, E., Carragher, M., O'Halloran, R., et al. (2024). Optimising healthcare communication for people with aphasia in hospital: Key directions for future research. *Current Physical Medicine and Rehabilitation Reports, 12,* 89–99. https://doi.org/10.1007/s40141-024-00431-z

Lerman, A., Goral, M., & Obler, L. K. (2020). The complex relationship between pre-stroke and post-stroke language abilities in multilingual individuals with aphasia. *Aphasiology, 34*(11), 1319–1340. https://doi.org/10.1080/0268703 8.2019.1673303

Loveall, S. J., Channell, M. M., Abbeduto, L., & Conners, F. A. (2019). Verb production by individuals with down syndrome during narration. *Research in Developmental Disabilities, 85*, 82–91.

Montembeault, M., Brambati, S. M., Gorno-Tempini, M. L., & Migliaccio, R. (2018). Clinical, anatomical, and pathological features in the three variants of primary progressive aphasia: A review. *Frontiers in Neurology, 9*, 338571.

Mooijman, S., Schoonen, R., Roelofs, A., & Ruiter, M. B. (2022). Executive control in bilingual aphasia: A systematic review. *Bilingualism: Language and Cognition, 25*(1), 13–28.

O'Halloran, R., Grohn, B., & Worrall, L. (2012). Environmental factors that influence communication for patients with a communication disability in acute hospital stroke units: A qualitative metasynthesis. *Archives of Physical Medicine and Rehabilitation, 93*(1), S77–S85.

O'Halloran, R., Renton, J., Harvey, S., McSween, M. P., & Wallace, S. J. (2024). Do social determinants influence post-stroke aphasia outcomes? A scoping review. *Disability and Rehabilitation, 46*(7), 1274–1287.

Paplikar, A., Mekala, S., Bak, T. H., Dharamkar, S., Alladi, S., & Kaul, S. (2019). Bilingualism and the severity of poststroke aphasia. *Aphasiology, 33*(1), 58–72.

Paradis, M., & Libben, G. (2014). *The assessment of bilingual aphasia.* Psychology Press.

Peñaloza, C., Barrett, K., & Kiran, S. (2020). The influence of prestroke proficiency on poststroke lexical-semantic performance in bilingual aphasia. *Aphasiology, 34*(10), 1223–1240. https://doi.org/10.1080/02687038.2019. 1666082

Ross, L. A., McCoy, D., Wolk, D. A., Coslett, H. B., & Olson, I. R. (2010). Improved proper name recall by electrical stimulation of the anterior temporal lobes. *Neuropsychologia, 48*(12), 3671–3674.

Sparing, R., Dafotakis, M., Hesse, M. D., & Fink, G. R. (2007). Enhancing language performance with transcranial direct current stimulation in healthy humans: Implications for rehabilitation and recovery of function after stroke. *Journal of Neurology, 254*, 65–65.

Smith, G., Janetti, B. B., Sarin, M., & Garraffa, M. (2023). Grammar in Adults with Neurodevelopmental Disorders: A Scoping Review from the Last 10 Years. *Languages, 8*(4), 248. https://doi.org/10.3390/languages8040248

Index